Narrative Based Health Care:
Sharing Stories
A multiprofessional workbook

Narrative Based Health Care:
Sharing Stories
A multiprofessional workbook

Trisha Greenhalgh
GP and Professor of Primary Care
UCL, Highgate Hill, London, UK

Anna Collard
Social Action for Health
London, UK

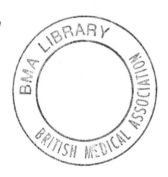

© BMJ Publishing Group 2003
BMJ Books is an imprint of the BMJ Publishing Group

First published by BMJ Books in 2003
by BMJ Books, BMA House, Tavistock Square,
London WC1H 9JR

www.bmjbooks.com

British Library Cataloguing in Publication Data

A catalogue record for this book is available from the British Library

ISBN 0 7279 1718 8

Typeset by SIVA Math Setters, Chennai, India
Printed and bound in Spain by GraphyCems, Navarra

Contents

Acknowledgements

The Diabetes Sharing Stories Project would not have been possible without the generous financial support of Diabetes UK, the enthusiastic participation of the group members, and input from the following individuals and organisations:

- Marcia Rigby (Administrator) and Jane Hughes (Research Fellow), Department of Primary Care and Population Studies, University College London
- John Eversley, Public Policy Research Unit, Queen Mary & Westfield College
- Elizabeth Bayliss and Staff (Myra Garrett, Shahanara Begum, Syed Shahriar) at Social Action for Health (previously Tower Hamlets Health Strategy Group)
- Akgul Baylav, Barbara James, Anjum Fareed (formerly locality/service coordinators) and Nirban Chowdhury (Health Promotion Adviser), East London & City Health Authority (ELCHA)
- Susan Harrison (formerly Primary Care Advocacy Manager); Marcia Wilson (Primary Care Advocacy Manager); Dilara Khan (Primary Care Advocacy Team Leader); Rowshanara Chowdhury (Parents Advisory Group), Tower Hamlets Healthcare Trust (THHT)
- Jane Bushby, Debbie James, Denise McEneaney (Maternity Services Managers); Professor Graham Hitman, Professor Peter Kopelman, Dr Barbara Boucher and Husneara Begum (Clinical Adult Diabetes Services), Royal London Hospitals Trust
- Sue Gardener (Head Continuing Learning), Urban Learning Foundation
- Mohamud Ahmed, Community Organisations Forum
- Tessa Griffith and Sayed Imran (Ethnic Health Advisers), Diabetes UK
- Dr Isabel Hodkinson (Diabetes Adviser) Tower Hamlets Primary Care Group
- Dr Anita Berlin (Senior Lecturer in Primary Health Care), Imperial College School of Medicine
- Sharif Islam (Research Fellow), Department of Dental Public Health, London Hospital Medical School

Introduction

About this workbook

The main theme of this workbook, as described in detail below, is how stories about illness can be used as the raw material for group learning and service development in the health professions. The workbook is itself a unique and contextual story – about how one group of health care workers, who worked with a particular ethnic group in a deprived inner city community, identified and attempted to meet their own learning needs and improve local services using the oral storytelling tradition. The workbook is designed to be used as an example of one group's journey, and not as the definitive last word on what all health professionals need to know about diabetes or how they should go about learning it!

There is no need to limit the storytelling technique to diabetes. We used diabetes as the basis for our own group work partly because it is particularly prevalent in the Bangladeshi community we were working with, and partly because our work was funded by the charity Diabetes UK. But the same storytelling technique can be used to address the clinical and service needs for any complex health problem which impacts on the lives of people, their families and communities. For this reason we have deliberately *not* provided a comprehensive list of references on diabetes at the end of each unit. Rather, we have provided examples of the type of further reading that a learner in an interprofessional study group might find useful.

Our aim in preparing this workbook was to provide a resource for individual reflection and group discussion. Please look through it, share it, talk about it, and use it to inspire your own unique response to training and service development in your area. We hope that the open-ended nature of the study units, the lists of further reading, and the range of suggestions for how to use the material in interactive group work, will allow participants, facilitators, and tutors to explore new ways of teaching and learning.

As we explain in this introduction, there are many unanswered questions about the use of storytelling in educating health professionals, promoting multiprofessional teamwork, or developing or modifying local services. We would be most interested in hearing about your own experiences with using stories in such circumstances. Please email us on *stories@pcps.ucl.ac.uk* with your own story! Meanwhile, there is no need to read the whole of this introduction before you get started – the main section of the book is self-explanatory on a practical level. However, if you are interested in the contextual background or theoretical basis for the work we did, you can return to this section at a later date.

About the Diabetes Sharing Stories Project

The stories, and fragments of stories, presented here are the work of ten health advocates[1] who were members of our first learning set and who participated in an experimental training programme in Tower Hamlets in late 2000. The original programme was part of the Diabetes Sharing Stories Project, which was set up to explore the educational potential of storytelling in improving the understanding and management of diabetes and health outcomes among adults with diabetes in the Bangladeshi community. The project was funded by Diabetes UK and builds on work done by a research team led by Trisha Greenhalgh at University College London (UCL).[2,3] As the project moved from a pure research phase to a development focus, the UCL team began to work in partnership with a voluntary sector organisation, Social Action for Health, to pilot new training methods for health professionals and new services for patients. The training programme for advocates subsequently led to the development of a number of advocate-led, group-based education and support sessions for people with diabetes in Tower Hamlets and neighbouring boroughs, some of which are now funded by mainstream Primary Care Organisations and acute trusts.

The exchange of stories, based on the experiences of working in the health services and with the local community, formed the focal point of each of the nine formal group workshops in the programme. Prior to the formal sessions, we held two informal "taster" workshops in which people could try out working in small groups and set priorities for topics to cover. After each of the group workshops, the participants wrote up a story and submitted it as part of their assessment for the course. A storytelling template (see Appendix), which aimed to encourage reflection and help the participants draw out their learning needs, was developed for this.

The stories produced by the advocates covered a wide range of themes, and each one has many different learning points. It was a difficult and somewhat artificial task to select particular ones to illustrate the different topic areas covered in the first course and reproduced in this workbook. As you will see, a lot of the stories cut across the different topic headings – which, of course, more accurately mirrors the reality of having diabetes or helping a person or a family with that condition.

In one respect, the stories presented in this workbook do not adequately reflect the richness of the stories told by word of mouth within the safety of the group, nor the discussions that followed and the learning gained through telling and listening to each other's stories. Even as fragments, however, they raise a wealth of issues and highlight important recurring themes. All of these are vital to understanding diabetes, its impact on families and individuals, its management and implications for health professionals and health services in any community, and the Bangladeshi community in particular.

We have reproduced the stories faithfully as they were written by the participants in our learning group, except where issues of confidentiality required us to change details that might identify a patient, client or relative of a group member. The participants in our group sessions were Arati Nath, Manwara Khatun, Umme Nessa (Royal London Hospitals Trust); Jakia Haque, Rafia Begum, Rashida Khatun, Hosna Begum, Shelly Das (Tower Hamlets Healthcare Trust); Nazeerah Rahman (Stepney Housing & Development Agency); and Waheeda Islam (St Dunstan's Bangladeshi Resource Centre).

Although this workbook is based on our first learning set (which focused entirely on the Bangladeshi community), we have subsequently run the same programme with health professionals and advocates from a wide range of ethnic groups including Chinese, Iranian, Turkish, Punjabi, Farsi, and Gujurati. We found that the storytelling format enabled participants from these different communities to highlight the commonalities as well as the contrasts in their professional experiences, and to learn generalisable lessons about interprofessional working and client support.

About storytelling

In this project, we were privileged to work with colleagues from the British Bangladeshi community, whose cultural heritage includes a rich narrative tradition within Bangladeshi literature, theatre, myth, legend, song, and dance. But as this section argues, we believe that communicating by storytelling is fundamental to the human experience, and is a powerful medium for communicating, learning, and problem solving in health and social care, whatever the language or culture.

The story as a linguistic form has a number of characteristics. In particular:[4]
- It runs through time – that is, it has a beginning, a series of unfolding events, and (we anticipate) an ending.
- It requires both a narrator and a listener, whose different viewpoints are brought to bear on how it is told.
- It involves selective reporting of particular details – the ones that are important to this version of the telling.
- It focuses on characters – what they do, and what happens to them.

- It includes an emotional dimension – that is, it is not just about what happens but how the characters *feel* about it.
- It has a plot – which gives meaning to unfolding events and provides continuity, emergence, unforeseen twists, and denouements.
- It invites an interpretation – and, if told in groups, promotes the dialogue of competing interpretations.

One of the first things medical students learn when they start their clinical training is how to "clerk a patient" – that is, record and present a patient's problem under a set of standard subheadings, beginning with Presenting Complaint and working through topics such as Past Medical History, Drug History and, finally, the Clinical Examination (divided into cardiovascular, respiratory, abdominal, genitourinary and so on). Anything that cannot be classified as a "fact" under these headings has no formal place in the medical record. Yet the complex, holistic, emotional, and relentlessly contextual illness experiences of patients lend themselves far better to the rich medium of storytelling than to the highly structured clinical clerking advocated by the medical curriculum.[5] Anthropologists Byron and Mary-Jo Good documented – somewhat disturbingly – that over the course of their undergraduate training, medical students are systematically socialised into standardising and sanitising the patient's narrative, and that they become progressively less aware of dimensions of the illness that are defined as "irrelevant" within the medical model.[6]

In the 1980s, doctors (especially psychiatrists) began to publish the unadulterated narratives of their patients,[7–9] perhaps partly as a backlash against the artificial format for "taking a history" imposed on them at medical school. Soon afterwards, "real" illness narratives published by the patients themselves[10–13] became popular both as general reading and for the education of health professionals. More recently, a major research collaboration has begun with the aim of systematically recording, indexing and publishing a wide collection of illness narratives using both text-based formats and video and internet technologies.[14]

A growing academic literature gives theoretical basis for what some doctors (and most patients) know intuitively – that narrative can be a more sophisticated tool for recording and analysing an illness than the conventional clinical clerking.[4,15–17] As one of us has previously argued:

> When doctors take a medical history, we inevitably act as ethnographers, historians, and biographers, requiring to understand aspects of personhood, personality, social and psychological functioning as well as biological and physical phenomena. ... The narrative provides meaning, context, and perspective for the patient's predicament. It defines how, why, and in what way he or she is ill. It offers, in short, a possibility of understanding which cannot be arrived at by any other means.[4]

Twenty years ago, such sentiments would have been rejected as either heretical or "woolly" by the mainstream medical profession. But in recent years, even such conventional publications as the *Journal of the American Medical Association* are now offering papers on "narrative competence":

> With narrative competence, physicians can reach and join their patients in illness, recognize their own personal journeys through medicine, acknowledge kinship with and duties toward other health care professionals, and inaugurate consequential discourse with the public about health care. By bridging the divides that separate physicians from patients, themselves, colleagues, and society, narrative medicine offers fresh opportunities for respectful, empathic, and nourishing medical care.[18]

Given the recent surge of interest in illness narratives, and the many anecdotal accounts of learning from such narratives,[19] it is perhaps surprising that the use of storytelling in the education of health and social care professionals has only recently been documented and evaluated.[20–22] Yet the health professions have a long and honourable tradition of storytelling. From the formal grand round and clinical case conference to the informal "corridor consultation",[23–25] and, in a different tradition, the Balint Groups in general practice,[26] doctors have discussed and compared patients' stories as a means of both learning more about the disease and solving particular clinical problems.

An emerging body of psychological research identifies the story in all its uniqueness and untidiness as the building block of clinical expertise. Medical students start by learning detailed "rules" about the cause, course and treatment of each clinical condition. As they gain knowledge they convert these rules to stereotypical stories ("illness scripts"). They refine their knowledge by accumulating atypical and alternative stories via experience and the oral tradition of sharing case histories. Furthermore, there is growing evidence that clinical knowledge is stored in doctors' memories *as stories* rather than as structured collections of abstracted facts.[23,27,28]

Kathryn Montgomery Hunter is a professor of literature who spent several years watching and listening to doctors going about their duties. As her detailed fieldwork showed, clinical decision-making occurs by the *selective* application of general rules to the unique predicament of particular individuals and contexts.[23,27] Hunter was struck that even though doctors often think of patients' storytelling as digression, stories are actually a surprisingly efficient way of compressing information. In her words: "Neither biology nor information science has improved upon the story as a means of ordering and storing the experience of human and clinical complexity. Neither is it likely to."[23] The examples given in this workbook illustrate the truth of this statement – some of the stories are as short as four or five lines, but they convey worlds of experience and suggest whole chapters of interpretations and potential ways forward.

McDrury and Alterio studied recent changes in the postgraduate education of nurses, for whom the telling of stories in educational settings traditionally took place in "informal space" (during coffee breaks and on the bus when travelling home), while the official nursing curriculum mainly comprised lists, formulae, and rules that had been deliberately detached and abstracted from any real life experiences.[20] Increasingly, however, stories are used formally and explicitly in nurse education, and comparable settings to the medical grand round are increasingly found. Drawing on previous theoretical work,[20,22] Alterio suggests a number of explicit advantages of the story in the education of health professionals (see Box).

Role of stories in the education of health professionals

- Convey information
- Express views
- Share experiences
- Entertain
- Connect with others
- Encourage cooperative activity
- Encompass holistic perspectives
- Value emotional realities
- Integrate subjective aspects of learning (feelings) with objective aspects (thoughts)
- Link theory to practice
- Stimulate students' critical thinking skills
- Capture complexities of situations
- Reveal multiple perspectives
- Make sense of experience
- Encourage self review
- Construct new knowledge

Reproduced with permission from Alterio[29]

There is no reason to assume that health professionals other than doctors and nurses build their knowledge any differently. Indeed, professions such as health advocates and linkworkers, who generally deal with complex cases – language and cultural barriers, the interface between health and social care, comorbidity, special needs, and extremes of age – presumably have *less* use for the structured clinical clerking and more use for the unique and highly personalised illness narrative. The illness experiences and health needs of all of us, and perhaps particularly those of minority ethnic groups, are inextricably bound up in the wider story of our lives within our family and social group. Medical anthropologist Vieda Skultans expresses this well:

> … the illness narrative of a patient tells at least two stories: the highly personal experience of the illness itself, embedded within a deeper narrative of social networks, folk models, mythology and cultural history. This second, cultural narrative may itself contain a story of society's struggle for health and wholeness in an alien world. Accounts from a migrant or colonised culture, for example, often describe a shared past or present experience of separation, loss, physical hardship, discrimination, poverty, and persecution, all of which may be crucially important influences upon the nature and course of the illness.[30]

Various stories related in this workbook illustrate this stories-within-stories phenomenon. The individual case history, personalised and contextualised within the wider family and social narrative, is thus a unique tool for crossing the cultural divide, exploring "otherness" (that is, experiencing worlds and identities that we can never know directly), and supporting a holistic approach to the complex and interrelated health, social, and cultural needs of vulnerable minority groups.

One word of warning. Although the use of stories in health care was considered poor science until relatively recently, the "narrative turn" is now becoming very popular and there is a great temptation to think that every problem has a story-shaped solution. Cox has argued that the story is not merely the unit of teaching ("the case") and the unit of analysis (the "case conference"), but also the unit of clinical memory (doctors and nurses learn about illnesses in storied form, and knowledge is stored in our memories *as* stories); he implicitly suggests that because the story is so memorable, so richly textured, and so interesting, we should abandon all other forms of communication, learning or analysis.[24] But as one of us has argued in a commentary on Cox's paper, storytelling may be better targeted where it has shown to have most "added value" – and specifically in four situations:[25]

- **Stories for exploring "otherness".** Research has shown how the storied approach is particularly suited to revealing worlds that are otherwise closed to us – such as those of the profoundly physically and mentally sick, the traumatised, displaced, or socially excluded; and people of different age, gender or ethnicity to ourselves.[1,5–8]

- **Stories for prompting the imagination.** Good clinical, moral, and practical judgements are not simply picked out of the sky. They arise from the same creative imagination that allows the scientist to generate worthwhile research hypotheses and the writer to develop a winning storyline or film script. The story is the ideal format for putting a range of options to a patient or client when the "right" decision is not self-evident ("If we did this you might find that such-and-such could happen, but if we did *that* instead you would have the option of so-and-so"). You will see from the template on p. 65 that in our own learning groups we explicitly asked "How could the story have ended differently?", and pursued this when considering changes in the service.
- **Stories for critical reflection on professional practice.** As health professionals, we not only tell stories about patients; we tell them about ourselves. Storytelling enables us to reflect on, uphold, and refine our roles as health professionals, especially in relation to critical or significant events. Given a protected small group environment, we tend to tell stories about "difficult" patients and situations, about our professional roles and perceived failures in them, and about contentious relationships within and across professional boundaries.[20] Stories potentially allow us to "get inside" the experience of other health professionals, clarify roles and responsibilities, and promote mutual understanding and respect. This is discussed further on p. xvi.
- **Stories as a research tool.** Recording and analysing the stories of patients and health professionals can provide key insights into beliefs, attitudes, behaviours and barriers to change. But be warned – the very fact that storytelling (like many other fundamental tools of qualitative research) is an aspect of ordinary human interaction means that there is a temptation for undertrained individuals to believe that they are adequately equipped to do research! In reality, the techniques for using storytelling as a *research* tool (such as discourse analysis or the use of sophisticated computer software to extract themes and develop theories) require extended training and are beyond the scope of this book but are covered by specialist research texts.[17]

If we move from the clinician–patient (or advocate–client) encounter to an analysis of health care (and social care) organisations, there is an important (though somewhat obscure) literature on how we can use stories to understand how such organisations work (or, more commonly, how they fail to work effectively or efficiently). For example, organisational anthropologists Czarniawska and Gabriel have separately shown how stories can illuminate the depths of organisational culture and highlight why a particular organisation (or subgroup within one) is so resistant to change.[31,32]

Buckler and Zien have explored the role of stories as catalysts for creativity in organisations. In an in-depth anthropological study of 11 highly successful companies from both the commercial and service sector, they showed that storytelling techniques were consistently (and sometimes explicitly) used to enable employees to break free of old ways of thinking and encourage innovation. In their words:

> [Through stories] senior people in innovative companies foster a sense of community and common purpose and thus create an environment that allows employees to explore new ideas and, if necessary, break the old rules. ... Storytelling offers a particularly evocative medium for articulating a [dynamic] vision. ... The most effective leaders continually reshape these stories to offer fresh insights, uncover new challenges, and reinforce the notion that every employee can and should contribute to their full potential.[33]

The notion that innovative thinking by definition involves "breaking the rules" is an important one. The UK National Health Service is the largest bureaucracy in the world (with the possible exception of Indian Railways), and whilst organisational change in the NHS is viewed as essential for modernisation,[34] it is increasingly acknowledged that such change is not easy to achieve in complex, rule-based organisations. If Buckler and Zien are correct, storytelling could be one medium through which health and social care staff (by giving particular stories a "different ending" that resonates with all stakeholders) will come to work effectively across boundaries and conceptualise a new and better service. The potential of a good story to "ignite action" in complex organisations is well described in the management literature,[35] and the technique of appreciative enquiry (AI) is increasingly being used by management consultants to achieve precisely this goal.[36]

It is conceivable (though arguably still a research hypothesis) that storytelling will enable interprofessional and interorganisational groups in health and social services not merely to compare experiences but to convert stories into action and construct the new service. Bate describes one such project in a hospital trust, in which stories were used first to delineate the problem, then to build a vision, and finally to drive action through what he calls an emerging "community of practice" across the organisation.[37]

In summary, the time is well overdue for the systematic use of storytelling as a means for gaining a holistic understanding of the patient's predicament, and in particular for identifying the full picture (physical, psychological, social, economic, and so on) of illness and its impact on the individual, the family, and the community. There is also evidence that storytelling can be used at an organisational level to draw disparate individuals and groups together and produce sustainable, patient-centred changes in services.

The literature on how best to use storytelling for such ambitious goals is still patchy, and at a research level there are many more questions than answers, some of which are currently being addressed by psychologists, anthropologists, social scientists, linguists, and others.[38] But there is already a consistent and clear message from research to date: that stories are simple yet powerful tools for achieving understanding, building a shared perspective on a problem, and catalysing change.

We believe that there is no "right" or "evidence-based" way to use storytelling either for supporting professional reflection, promoting interprofessional working, or developing health services, though there are some established principles for effective adult learning and for working in groups (see below). Perhaps it is time for us all to "just do it" and see how storytelling works for our own local context and priorities.

About learning in groups

The rise in popularity of group work in educational settings[39] has paralleled the development of new theories of learning. Traditional instructivist learning theories depict learning in terms of the accumulation of facts, like storing money in a bank, and assume that learning can be assessed by the reproduction of these facts. Behaviourist theories, also part of the "old school" of pedagogy, depict learning in terms of performance outputs, like teaching a dog to beg for a reward, and which deny – or at least, refuse to analyse – any key role of consciousness in the learning process. Educationalists are replacing these conceptual frameworks with theories based on *experiential learning, informal (tacit) learning*, and the *social construction of knowledge*.

Experiential approaches to teaching and learning assume that facts are not fixed and immutable elements of thought but are constantly formed and re-formed through reflection and experience. Learning is seen as a continuous process in which every new experience builds on, and integrates with, the accumulated experiences that have gone before. Social discourse – that is, discussion with colleagues – is a crucial means of consolidating or changing understanding.

The experiential learning cycle developed by Lewin (and popularised by Kolb)[40] associated with conventional theories of adult learning does not explicitly incorporate the role of the group. As depicted in the Figure, the link between reflection and the formation of new abstract concepts is a highly individual one that carries the risk of a limited frame of reference and "navel gazing".

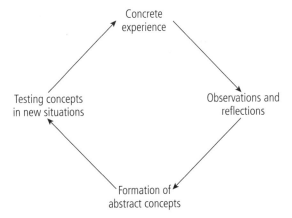

The experiential learning cycle (Lewin and Kolb)

The potential downside of group work for individual learning is groupthink (a shared sense of unanimity, invulnerability, and moral blindness in which poor decisions are irrationally produced and fiercely defended by a group unconsciously avoiding conflict),[39,41] and which a skilled facilitator must take steps to guard against.

Potential impact of small group work on experiential learning

- Encourages learners to control and direct their learning
- Enables learners to identify gaps in their understanding and make connections between concepts
- Activates previously acquired understanding
- Promotes questioning and discussion
- Promotes higher level activities conducive to deep learning (such as analysis, synthesis, critical reflection) rather than surface learning activities (memorisation, recollection and reproduction)
- Allows application and development of ideas
- Promotes change in attitudes and motivation
- Improves confidence and self-esteem
- Promotes transformational learning – that is, application of existing knowledge to new situations and subsequent reframing of knowledge and concepts[42]

Informal learning is, as the name implies, learning through informal and unofficial channels, and often when unaware that learning is taking place at all. The distinction between formal (explicit) and informal (tacit) knowledge is illustrated by the new university graduate who despite a long list of qualifications is unable to do the job. What such an individual needs is not more knowledge but some practical "know-how" of the kind that in days gone by was often provided by a long period of apprenticeship.

The world of work (especially that of health professionals) generally involves complex fields of practice, in which items of knowledge are influenced to some extent by one another but do not have simple, linear connections (for example, we know that a person with poorly controlled diabetes will probably develop an acute crisis at some stage but we cannot say precisely what or when). Learning that builds capability and know-how in these situations occurs when individuals engage with new and unfamiliar contexts in a meaningful and reflective way. The young doctor (or new parent) who tries to prepare for all eventualities by reading the textbook will find that the practical wisdom of experience cannot be learnt by theory or rote. Rather, such a stage is reached through a *transformation* process in which existing knowledge and skills are adapted and tuned to the new circumstances.[42]

The three key factors that promote transformational learning are:[42]
- **feedback** to the learner about the impact of their actions and those of others
- **reflection** by the learner on the meaning of their actions and the feedback received, and
- **planned change** in behaviour in response to feedback and reflection.

It is well established that reflective learners are receptive to feedback and able to adapt appropriately, whilst poor learners are either unreceptive to feedback or adapt inappropriately.[43,44] Reflective learners transform as the world around them changes; poor learners simply complain about it. The role of the group in transformational learning is clear: by hearing the story of an aspect of professional practice, and providing honest, considered and curious feedback, the group can encourage and support reflection and share in the construction of possible different "endings" to the story.[42] Dr Anita Berlin (personal communication, July 2000) has modified Kolb's single-loop learning cycle, shown in the Figure below. Discourse with others increases the chance that reflection will lead to new and transformed meaning for the individual. This transformational potential is the "added value" of group discussion over and above individual reflection. In addition, of course, group work enhances motivation and provides a social setting and practical context for the material learnt – all critical components of adult learning.[45]

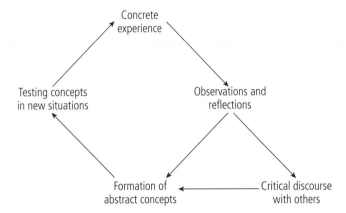

Effect of group work on the experiential learning cycle (Berlin)

This is the theoretical basis for the increasing variety of group-based initiatives in continuing professional development, including:

- Group-assisted reflection techniques, in which learners simply describe recent cases and identify (for example) "patients' unmet needs" (PUNs) and "doctor's educational needs" (DENs).[46] The presence of the group is not critical to the technique but as described above can greatly enhance its effectiveness.
- Small group, problem-based learning, in which a case scenario forms the basis of an exploratory, tutor-facilitated dialogue and emerging action plan by a group of participants.[47]
- Collective learning sets, which are intended to "create the atmosphere and use the processes that stimulate learning from action". The actions take place outside the set meeting and often away from other set members. The set provides the focus for the reflective part of the cycle, leading to learning from experience and the formation of plans informed by this learning.[48]
- Critical incident analysis, in which a disaster or near-miss forms the basis of an interprofessional review of structures and systems in small group format, with a view to identifying modifiable problems and implementing change. Originally developed for analysing in-flight emergencies,[49] the technique was adapted to a clinical context and renamed significant event audit.[50,51]

The learning group described in the rest of this workbook had features of all the above approaches. In the early stages, much of the time was spent on reflective activities and problem-based learning scenarios elicited and directed by the authors (T.G. and A.C.), who took on the role of tutors. But as the group developed and people's knowledge and confidence increased, the predominant model became that of a learning set and the authors acted more as facilitators. As you might imagine, on occasions when one group member brought a critical story (such as a death, a near-miss, or other profoundly upsetting incident), the group operated more in critical incident mode.

One final dimension of group work is its particular suitability for interprofessional working. The greater the range of perspectives and disciplines represented in the group, the greater the range of interpretive feedback that can be provided to the individual learner and the greater the potential for changes in attitudes and motivation. The use of facilitated group work for building teams and promoting interprofessional working is covered in detail elsewhere.[52–55] Given that both group work *and* storytelling are both established techniques for breaking down interprofessional boundaries, the potential for storytelling *in interprofessional groups* is potentially an extremely powerful tool for interorganisational change. We were disappointed that the core membership of our learning group included a relatively narrow range of professionals, but on several occasions we invited guests from the lay public (patients, carers) or other professions (diabetes specialist nurse, dietician, fitness officer, podiatrist, social worker, diabetologist) who joined the group and contributed very productively to discussions.

In summary, group work is a particularly effective method for supporting deep learning, multidisciplinary learning and interprofessional working. Group work encourages effective, transformational learning because it provides feedback in a supportive social context and promotes (indeed, requires) the activities of listening, questioning, explaining, comparing, consolidating, summarising, and evaluating.

Group work objectives

We know from experience that small group work tends to be fun, exhausting, and effective. To make it more fun, less exhausting, and more effective, we suggest some tips (which are all explained in more detail in a specialist textbook).[39]

1. **Get to know each other** before you start – including:
   - What are our names, professional backgrounds, and interests?
   - What relevant skills, experience or perspectives do individual members have?
   - What were our individual objectives in coming on the course and/or joining the group?

   All this may be done via a structured group exercise, but it is often easier and less stressful to allow people to chat informally for half an hour on arrival.

"Ice breaking" exercises often feel contrived and artificial, whereas everyone knows how to put the kettle on!

2. **Set some ground rules** – such as:
   - When will each session start and finish? How important is it that we all turn up to every session, and that we start and finish on time? How will we cope with members who turn up late or irregularly?
   - How will we run each session? Will members take it in turns to present or lead sessions? How about presenting in pairs?
   - How will we deal with interruptions and distractions (for example, latecomers, "bleeps", mobile phones, people "just popping out")?
   - How will we use our designated tutor or facilitator (if we have one)? If we don't have one, should one of us take on that role?
   - What methods (such as formal presentations, informal discussions, role play) and technologies (flip chart, video, computer etc.) will we use for our learning?
   - Do we have a specific task to complete (for example, a project to do) that has been set by someone outside the group, and if so, what are our terms of reference towards that individual or funding body?

We advise you to record your ground rules on flip chart paper and revisit them from time to time as your group develops and (perhaps) changes its priorities.

3. **Be aware of two aspects of the learning**
   - **Content** – that is, what is being covered. What is the clinical topic, what dimension of the problem is the focus of discussion, what depth is it being covered in, etc.?
   - **Process** – that is, how it is being covered. Who is speaking, who is listening (and who isn't), are any points of view being unreasonably dismissed, is the speaker simply stating their opinion or offering reasoned argument, etc.?

Attention to the group process is a crucial skill, which is covered in detail elsewhere.[39] It helps enormously to have a trained facilitator (process expert) as well as a content expert and for all members of the group to have read the basics of how groups work.

4. **Have a broad structure** in mind for every session. For example:
   - Set the agenda for the session (leaving time for practical things such as shifting furniture, moving to break-out rooms, and refreshments, as well as the other tasks listed below).
   - Agree on the topic to be covered, the methods to be used, the roles of the group members and tutor, and the learning objectives.
   - Run the session, modifying the objectives as you go along if necessary (for example, if it emerges that they were unrealistic).

- Evaluate this session.
- Plan the next session.

Again, these topics are covered in more detail in specialist books on group work,[39] but you will find the same principles in any good textbook on teaching and learning.

5. **Establish, and follow, rules for giving feedback**. For example:
   - Timing
     - Allocate protected time during or after the session for feedback
     - Try to give feedback as soon after the event as possible.
   - Packaging. When giving negative feedback:
     - Use the "criticism sandwich" – begin and end your feedback on a positive note (for example, "It was a good idea to try a role play here. Unfortunately I felt my brief was ambiguous, and I think quite a few others felt the same. As a result I felt the session didn't hang together. But still, we all got to know each other better and we've learnt some lessons for next time.")
     - Use "I" and give your experience of the behaviour (for example, "When you said …, I felt that you were … ").
   - Content
     - Stick to one or two points
     - Confine your comments to things that can be changed. There is no point saying "You've got an awful sense of humour", but you could say, "I felt it was inappropriate to make a joke at that point in your presentation"
     - Describe specific behaviours and give examples (for example, "You stood up and spoke loudly") rather than assigning motives ("You were trying to intimidate her")
     - Suggest alternative behaviours (for example, "Perhaps you could have asked everyone at that point if they were still with you").
   - Self awareness
     - Remember that feedback says a lot about you as well as about the person to whom it is directed
     - Ask yourself, "Why am I giving this feedback?" If you want to show how much you know, or contribute generally to the topic under discussion, the feedback session is not the place to do it.

6. **Include group skills as an explicit learning objective**
   The ability to work effectively in a group or team is important in itself, whatever the content of the group work. In addition to the diabetes-specific learning objectives described in the individual study units, this course is designed to provide training in the knowledge, skills, and attitudes needed to learn from, and contribute to, small group work in any context.

The objectives given in the Tables below are intended to be generalisable to any training course for health and health-related professions that involves storytelling in groups. We have expressed them in terms of two different levels recognised by an established further education provider (the London Open College Network, or LOCN, Levels 2 and 3) to take account of different achievement levels in different group members.

Notes and references

1 The term "advocate" is used generically to include all those involved in the training: primary care advocates and maternity services advocates from the Royal London Hospital, linkworkers or nursing support workers and community advocates or development workers. In all, ten advocates followed the programme described in this book.

2 Greenhalgh T, Chowdhury AM, Helman C. Health beliefs and folk models of diabetes in British Bangladeshis: a qualitative study. *BMJ* 1998;**316**:978–83.

3 Chowdhury AM, Helman C, Greenhalgh T. Food beliefs and practices in British Bangladeshis with diabetes: an ethnographic analysis. *Med Anthropol* 2000;**7**:209–26.

4 Greenhalgh T, Hurwitz B. Why study narrative? In: Greenhalgh T, Hurwitz B, eds. *Narrative-based medicine: dialogue and discourse in clinical practice*. London: BMJ Publishing Group, 1998: ch. 1, pp. 3–16.

5 Greenhalgh T. Narrative based medicine in an evidence-based world. In: Greenhalgh T, Hurwitz B, eds. *Narrative-based medicine: dialogue and discourse in clinical practice*. London: BMJ Publications, 1998: ch. 24, pp. 247–65.

6 Good B, Good M-J. Fiction and historicity in doctors' stories. In: Mattingly C, Garro L, eds. *Narrative and the cultural construction of illness and healing*. Berkeley, CA: University of California Press, 2000.

7 Sacks O. *The man who mistook his wife for a hat*. New York: Harper & Row, 1985.

8 Brody H. *Stories of sickness*. New Haven, CT: Yale University Press, 1987.

9 Kleinmann A. *The illness narratives: suffering, healing and the human condition*. New York: Basic Books, 1988.

10 Armstrong L. *It's not about the bike*. New York: Yellow Jersey Press, 2001.

11 Bauby J-D. *The diving bell and the butterfly*. London: Fourth Estate, 1998.

12 Diamond J. *C: because cowards get cancer too*. London: Vermillion Books, 1998.

13 Frank A. *At the will of the body: perspectives on illness. Boston*: Houghton–Mifflin, 1991.

14 Herxheimer A, McPherson A, Miller R, Shepperd S, Yahpe J, Ziebland S. Database of patients' experiences (DIPEx): a multi-media approach to sharing experiences and information. *Lancet* 2000;**355**:1540–3.

15 Mattingly C. *Healing dramas and clinical plots: the narrative structure of experience*. New York: Cambridge University Press, 1998.

16 Frank A. *The wounded storyteller: body, illness, and ethics*. Chicago: University of Chicago Press, 1995.

17 Riessman CK. *Narrative analysis*. Newbury Park, CA: Sage, 1993.

18 Charon R. The patient–physician relationship. Narrative medicine: a model for empathy, reflection, profession, and trust. *JAMA* 2001;**286**:1897–902.

19 Macnaughton J. Anecdote in clinical practice. In: Greenhalgh T, Hurwitz B, eds. *Narrative-based medicine: dialogue and discourse in clinical practice*. London: BMJ Publications, 1998: ch. 20, pp. 202–11.

20 McDrury L, Alterio M. *Learning through storytelling: using reflection and experience in higher education contexts*. Palmerston North: Dunmore Press, 2002.

21 McEwan H, Egan K. *Narrative in teaching, learning and research*. New York: Teachers College, Columbia University, 1995.

22 Witherell C, Nodding M, eds. *Stories lives tell: narrative and dialogue in education*. New York: Teachers College Press, 1991.

23 Hunter KM. *Doctors' stories*. Princeton, NJ: Princeton University Press, 1991.

24 Cox K. Stories as case knowledge: case knowledge as stories. *Med Educ* 2001; **35**:862–6.

25 Greenhalgh T. Storytelling should be targeted where it is known to have greatest added value. *Med Educ* 2001;818–19.

26 Rabin S, Maoz B, Elata-Alster G. Doctors' narratives in Balint groups. *Br J Med Psychol* 1999;**72**:121–5.

27 Hunter K. "Don't think zebras": uncertainty, interpretation, and the place of paradox in clinical education. *Theoret Med* 1996;**17**:225–41.

28 Eraut M. Non-formal learning, implicit learning and tacit knowledge. In: Coffield F, ed. *Informal learning*. Bristol: The Policy Press, 1999.

29 Alterio MG. Using storytelling to enhance student learning. Online paper, Institute for Learning and Teaching in Higher Education, Members' Resource Area, www.ilt.ac.uk, 2002.

30 Skultans V. Anthropology and narrative. In: Greenhalgh T, Hurwitz B, eds. *Narrative based medicine: dialogue and discourse in clinical practice*. London: BMJ Publications, 1998, pp. 225–32.

31 Czarniawska, B. *Narrating the organization. Dramas of institutional identity*. Chicago: University of Chicago Press, 1997.

32 Gabriel Y. *Storytelling in organisations: facts, fictions and fantasies*. Oxford: Oxford University Press, 2000.

33 Buckler SA, Zien KA. The spirituality of innovation: learning from stories. *J Product Innov Mngmnt* 1996;**13**:391–405.

34 Department of Health. *The NHS Plan*. London: NHS Executive, 2001.

35 Denning S. *The springboard: how storytelling ignites action in knowledge-era organisations*. New York: Butterworth–Heinemann, 2001.

36 Cooperrider D, Sorensen P, Yaeger TF, Whitney D, eds. *Appreciative enquiry: an emerging direction for organization development*. Champaign, IL: Stipe Publishing, 2001.

37 Bate SP. Towards a new form of politics in organisational change efforts: an anthropological case study of an emerging 'community of practice' within the UK Health Service. *Intervention. Journal of Culture, Organisation and Management*. In press.

38 See, for example, the archives of the academic discussion list narrative-health-research at www.jiscmail.ac.uk.

39 Elwyn G, Greenhalgh T, Macfarlane F. *Groups: a hands-on guide to small group work in health care, education, management and research*. Oxford: Radcliffe Medical Press, 2000.

40 Kolb DA. The process of experiential learning. In: Thorpe M, Edwards R, Hanson A. *Culture and processes of adult learning.* London: Routledge, 1993, pp. 138–56.

41 Janis IL. *Victims of groupthink.* Boston: Houghton–Mifflin, 1972.

42 Fraser S, Greenhalgh T. Coping with complexity: educating for capability. *BMJ* 2001;**323**:799–803.

43 Hull C. *Principles of behavior.* New York: Appleton–Century–Crofts, 1943.

44 Thorndike E. *The fundamentals of learning.* New York: Teachers College Press, 1932.

45 Lave J, Wenger E. *Situated learning: legitimate peripheral participation.* Cambridge: Cambridge University Press, 1990.

46 Eve R. Learning with PUNs and DENs – a method for determining educational needs and the evaluation of its use in primary care. *Educ Gen Pract* 2000;**11**:73–9.

47 Bligh J. Problem-based, small group learning. *BMJ* 1995;**311**:342–3.

48 McGill I, Beaty L. *Learning: a practitioner's guide.* London: Kogan Page, 1992.

49 Robinson LA, Stacy R, Spencer JA, Bhopal RS. How to do it: use facilitated case discussions for significant event auditing. *BMJ* 1995;**311**:315–18. (Available in full text on http://bmj.com/cgi/content/full/311/7000/315.)

50 Flanaghan J. The critical incident technique. *Psychol Bull* 1954;**51**:327–58.

51 Kemppainen JK. The critical incident technique and nursing care quality research *J Adv Nurs* 2000;**32**:1264–71.

52 Gorman P. *Managing multidisciplinary teams in the NHS.* London: Kogan Page, 1998.

53 Pritchard P, Pritchard J. *Teamwork for primary and shared care: a practical workbook,* 2nd edn. Oxford: Oxford Medical Publications, 1994.

54 Øvretveit J. *Organising multidisciplinary community teams.* HCS Working Paper. Brunel University: BIOSS: Uxbridge, 1986.

55 Øvretveit J. *Coordinating community care.* Open University Press: Milton Keynes, 1993.

Learning objectives for Level 2 LOCN credits: "Storytelling in group learning in health and care".

By the end of the course the learner will be expected to	The learner has demonstrated the ability to	Key assessment criteria	Key assessment evidence
1. Function effectively as a member of a professional learning group	(a) Set and apply ground rules (b) Agree group objectives for each session (c) Communicate information and feelings to the group (d) Respond appropriately and sensitively to information and feelings conveyed by other group members	Tutor observation of group process	Tutor report on performance in group
2. Understand and apply storytelling techniques in the context of group learning of health care professionals	(a) Select and share stories about the illness experience and health care encounters of clients in a protected group setting with fellow health professionals (b) Reflect on the perspectives and needs of clients as illustrated by stories shared in this professional setting (c) Show understanding of the role of emotions and life narrative in determining health behaviour	Tutor observation of group process Written accounts of clients' illness and life narratives showing relevance to topic area and sensitivity to clients' perspectives	Tutor report on performance in group Written accounts of clients' illness and life narratives following template or otherwise
3. Identify and address their own professional learning needs through storytelling in a professional group	(a) Identify own professional learning needs based on clients' stories of illness and health care encounters	Written account of clients' illness and life narratives	Identification of specific unmet learning needs arising from accounts of clients' illness and life narratives
4. Apply the information gained from storytelling to the development of health promotion materials	(a) Assist in the development of health promotion materials based on the needs identified through clients' illness and life narratives and the information collected to meet those needs	Tutor assessment of relevance, accuracy and validity of health promotion materials produced or co-produced by learner	Health promotion materials (written or otherwise) produced or co-produced by learner
5. Review own practice and record and report appropriately	(a) Produce written accounts of clients' illness and life narratives according to a structured template	Written accounts of clients' illness and life narratives Student self audit of explicit learning goals Tutor assessment of relevance, scope, and quality of written accounts of clients' illness and life narratives	Tutor report Witness testimony Personal action plan

Learning objectives for Level 3 LOCN credits: "Storytelling in group learning in health and care".

By the end of the course the learner will be expected to	The learner has demonstrated the ability to	Key assessment criteria	Key assessment evidence
1. Function effectively as a member of a professional learning group	(a) Set and apply ground rules (b) Agree group objectives for each session (c) Communicate information and feelings to the group (d) Respond appropriately and sensitively to information and feelings conveyed by other group members (e) Use a range of communication methods appropriately in group work (f) Evaluate each session in terms of both content and process	Tutor observation of group process	Tutor report on performance in group
2. Understand and apply storytelling techniques in the context of group learning of health care professionals	(a) Select and share stories about the illness experience and health care encounters of clients in a protected group setting (b) Reflect on the perspectives and needs of clients as illustrated by stories shared in this professional setting (c) Show understanding of the role of emotions and life narrative in determining health behaviour (d) Develop strategies to take account of these when supporting particular clients	Tutor observation of group process Written accounts of clients' illness and life narratives showing relevance to topic area, sensitivity to clients' perspectives, and suggestions for modification of professional input	Tutor report on performance in group Written account of clients' illness and life narratives following template or otherwise
3. Identify and address their own professional learning needs through storytelling in a professional group	(a) Identify own professional learning needs based on clients' stories of illness and health care encounters (b) Access and select information and resources to meet particular needs	Written account of clients' illness and life narratives showing awareness of learning needs arising from these accounts	Written account of clients' illness and life narratives
4. Use external sources to meet identified learning needs	(a) Access and select information and resources to meet particular needs	Tutor assessment of relevance, accuracy and validity of information and resources collected by learner	Annotated list of resources used and materials collected by learner

(Continued)

(Continued)

By the end of the course the learner will be expected to	The learner has demonstrated the ability to	Key assessment criteria	Key assessment evidence
5. Apply the information gained from storytelling to the development of health promotion materials	(a) Develop health promotion materials based on the needs identified through clients' illness and life narratives and the information collected to meet those needs	Assessment of relevance, accuracy and validity of health promotion materials produced or co-produced by learner	Health promotion materials (written or otherwise) produced or co-produced by learner
6. Review own practice and record and report appropriately	(a) Produce written accounts of clients' illness and life narratives that include sensitivity to clients' perspectives, a reflective interpretation and specific learning points	Tutor assessment of relevance, scope, quality and reflective interpretation of clients' illness and life narratives	Tutor report Witness testimony Personal action plan
	(b) Set appropriate and measurable goals for own learning and development based on these accounts	Student self audit of learning goals based on the above	

Unit 1
Learning about diabetes care – where should we start?

Background

Diabetes can affect any person of any age. It can involve almost every part of the body and its successful management requires attention to many different aspects of a person's lifestyle and health care. It is often hard to know where to start learning about diabetes, or how to select a manageable topic to study without losing a holistic, patient-focused approach to diabetes in general.

Suggested aim for this session

To explore the range and scope of the problems associated with diabetes.

Suggested learning objectives for this session

By the end of this session, participants should be able to:

- tell a story about a person with diabetes that includes all the aspects given in the template in the Appendix (p. 65)
- give examples of how diabetes affects the lives of patients, families, and carers
- give examples of the input of different health professionals to the care of people with diabetes
- identify and prioritise areas for further study.

Suggestions for group exercises

When you have read the story in the Box, try one or more of the following:

1. Discuss the story of Mrs Begum. Brainstorm on a flipchart the different issues it raises about the care of people with diabetes. You should be able to come up with at least ten different areas for further exploration.
2. Divide your large group (if necessary) into smaller groups of about four people. Everyone in the group should have an opportunity to tell a story relating to the care of diabetes. Examples of stories you might share in this first session include:
   - a story about your own attempt to care for a person with diabetes;
   - a story about a friend or relative with diabetes;
   - a story about a patient or client with particular needs.

You may include anything you feel is relevant, but the aim of this session is to highlight aspects of your learning needs to explore more fully in future sessions.

3. When everyone in each small group has shared a story, reconvene in your larger group and share one or two examples of stories that demonstrate different learning needs for yourselves and other health professionals.

4. Reconvene in your small groups and make sure each group has a stack of "Post-it" notes. Write ONE potential training topic on each note. Keep doing this until you can think of no more topics. By the end, you should have 40 or 50 Post-its, each with a different topic. Now, sort them into themes so that you fill the number of slots allocated to your course.

(In our first Sharing Stories course we had a total of 12 sessions, including two introductory and planning sessions and a final plenary. In the first two sessions we learned about group work and produced the list of topics we have used to structure this book by means of this Post-it exercise.)

Suggested assignment

Write up a story about a person with diabetes in the first person, that is, *as if it were you*. It should be based on the experience of a real person – a relative, a patient or client, or even yourself if you have diabetes! Start the story "My name is X and I have diabetes. This is about how the illness affects my life, and about my hopes and fears."

When you have done this, identify three things that health professionals might need to learn in order to help the person better.

Further reading

A guide to small group work

Elwyn G, Greenhalgh T, Macfarlane F. *Groups: a hands-on guide to small group work in health care, education, management and research.* Oxford: Radcliffe Medical Press, 2000.

A general guide to diabetes care

Mackinnon M. *Providing diabetes care in general practice: a practical guide for the primary health care team*, 4th edition. London: Class Publishing, 2002. See in particular Part 1 (ch. 1–3), pp. 3–38.

A patient with complex needs

Mrs Begum is 60 years old, and is a newly diagnosed diabetic on insulin. She is lonely, with multiple illnesses. She lives with her 85-year-old husband.

Mrs Begum became hospitalised to stabilise her diabetes and treatment. There was a language barrier, which resulted in a poor assessment of her needs. Consequently her diabetic condition deteriorated on discharge back home. For example, her loneliness increased and she became incapable of providing self-care due to her other illnesses and her mobility became restricted. Mrs Begum strongly felt that her previous conditions had given rise to her diabetes.

Mrs Begum's husband, who is also ailing, felt dissatisfied with the care given and distressed because he was unable to provide appropriate support. This led to friction between husband and wife. Social services also felt helpless because of the poor communication. Mrs Begum was not adopting a healthy lifestyle. That is, she had poor eating patterns, poor nutrition, poor standards of hygiene, and lack of exercise. These resulted in a diabetic crisis.

Why did you choose this story?

Mrs Begum has multiple illnesses and has recently been diagnosed with diabetes but has no support.

Could anything have been done differently?

- Provision of an interpreter for the patient at the hospital
- Caring assistants at home to provide health care and monitor Mrs Begum's needs
- Education for patient on her drug administration
- Home help to maintain home hygiene
- Social services to arrange for safety equipment.

What questions or issues does this story raise?

The story raises the issue of resource allocation and equal access to services. It also identifies the need for diabetic support and referrals, for example, a diabetic support group. The need for an interpreter/advocate cannot be emphasised enough.

What are the learning points?

- Understanding of diabetes and its signs and symptoms
- Ability to give own drugs and amount of insulin needed in accordance with blood sugar levels
- Hence, need to be able to carry out urine and blood testing
- Patient has to understand her dietary needs.

In my opinion this patient did not appear to have fully understood her condition since she showed a poor grasp of diabetes. This therefore raises the need for a domiciliary linkworker to work with both patients and professionals in helping the patient to understand the diabetic condition and provide feedback on the patient's progress to the health professionals.

Tutor's comment

Like many people with diabetes, this elderly patient has complex needs for which there are no simple solutions, compounded by lack of adequate assessment. Input from both health and social care professionals, and from lay support groups, could help her considerably. But where to start? The complexity of the problem highlights the fact that patients' unmet needs often reflect professionals' own learning needs. A systematic list of all her problems is needed in the first instance. (The use of a multidisciplinary team of professionals to address patients' complex needs is dealt with in more detail in Unit 9.)

Unit 2
The diagnosis of diabetes

Background

It is said that diabetes is no longer a death sentence but it is still a life sentence. Appropriate management at the time of diagnosis, and during the difficult months that follow, can turn a disaster story into a coping story. Conversely, lack of understanding of the patient's concerns, lack of explanation, and lack of planning can set the stage for a lifelong tragedy.

Suggested aim for this session

For participants to explore the experiences and concerns of newly diagnosed patients with diabetes and identify areas that should be covered in both education and clinical management.

Suggested learning objectives for this session

By the end of this session, participants should be able to:

* describe the common symptoms of new diabetes
* empathise with a patient who has recently been diagnosed with the condition
* assist in the preparation of a multidisciplinary care plan for such a patient
* provide aspects of this care plan appropriate to their own professional background.

Suggestions for group exercises

When you have read the story in the Box, try one or more of the following:

1. Discuss the stories of Mrs Iqbal and Mr Ahmed. Discuss what you would say to each of them (a) at the time the diagnosis is given and (b) within one month of diagnosis.
2. If your group is multidisciplinary, share the different perspectives of different professionals on the patient's needs at diagnosis. You will probably find that doctors, nurses, dieticians, midwives, pharmacists, and health advocates all have different priorities, and that the priorities of those in a primary health care setting differ from those in specialist settings. You should not try to reach agreement on what is the "correct" way to manage the early period, but you should all try to understand and value the different perspectives of your colleagues.

3. Invite a person with diabetes to visit your group and tell you all what it was like when he or she was diagnosed. If he or she is now coping well, ask what helped them to achieve this. If there are now problems, ask the patient to suggest what could have been done differently.

Suggested assignment

Make a copy of the table below and complete it in relation to a particular patient or client who has recently been diagnosed with diabetes:

How the person found out they had diabetes	How they felt when they found out	Their initial beliefs, hopes, and fears about diabetes	What aspect of their early care could have been better, and how

Further reading

A guide to the symptoms of diabetes for health professionals
MacKinnon M. *Providing diabetes care in general practice: a practical guide for the primary health care team*, 4th edition. London: Class Publishing, 1998. (See Chapter 5, "The symptoms of diabetes", pp. 55–72.)

A guide to the symptoms of diabetes for patients
Understanding diabetes – a guide to diabetes for newly diagnosed patients and their families. Available free from Diabetes UK, 10 Parkway, London NWI 7AA; Tel 020 7323 1531; Fax 020 7637 3644; Email info@diabetes.org.uk, and downloadable from the website below.

Diabetes UK website – for professionals and the public
http://www.diabetes.org.uk/

Alternative Diabetes website – intended mainly for the public
This website has many ideas about living with diabetes and has a non-medical focus on lifestyle without being anti-medicine. http://www.alternativediabetes.com

The story of Mrs Iqbal

Mrs Iqbal was told she had developed diabetes. She was pregnant. She had to inject herself with insulin. After the pregnancy, Mrs Iqbal was put on tablets to control her diabetes. Mrs Iqbal was very scared when she learned she had diabetes. She felt that somehow the condition would "handicap" her. She didn't really understand what caused the diabetes. Her strongest emotion was fear. Mrs Iqbal, however, never developed a handicap and now leads a normal life.

Why did you choose this story?
I witnessed the reactions first hand.

Could anything have been done differently?
The causes of diabetes could have been better explained by those in the medical profession. Also Mrs Iqbal needed more reassurance than she received.

What questions or issues does this story raise?
Many people don't understand what diabetes is about. Also many horror stories tend to be passed around which cause fear.

What are the learning points?
People fear the unknown. If it can be explained to them what diabetes is about, it can help dispel fears.

The story of Mr Ahmed

Mr Ahmed is 60 years old and suffers from asthma. He is quite a big person. Recently, he went to see his GP because he thought he might have diabetes. He was passing a lot of urine. He was feeling drowsy most of the time and when he went shopping he felt breathless. The GP did a urine test and it showed glucose in Mr Ahmed's urine. The GP gave him advice on keeping to a good diet and told him to have regular check-ups with the nurse.

Mr Ahmed was very upset and worried about his diagnosis. He thought he would not be able to eat what he wanted to and was very anxious about whether he would be on tablets or put on insulin. Mr Ahmed kept going to the nurse for tests. He seemed to be going too much and he was not concentrating on what the GP had told him.

Could anything have been done differently?
Mr Ahmed should have been referred to a dietician. He needed someone to explain diabetes to him better, to reassure him that he could reduce his sugar intake, to tell him that he was safe and that the diabetes wouldn't affect his whole lifestyle.

What questions or issues does this story raise?
Mr Ahmed was very lost. He needed to speak to someone else suffering from diabetes. He needed to understand the diabetes better.

What are the learning points?
Mr Ahmed needed to see a dietician. He needed support and someone to monitor his diet.

Tutor's comment
These simple stories encapsulate two of the common hallmarks of the newly diagnosed patient – ignorance, and fear of the unknown. As the narrators rightly state, many people's only previous experience of diabetes is vague "horror stories" of blindness, amputation, and premature death. Both the patients described here need a structured programme of education and support tailored to their particular needs and choices.

Unit 3
Diabetes in the family

Background
Diabetes, particularly type 2, has a strong hereditary component. In some communities, particularly South Asian ethnic groups, it is extremely common and several members of a family may suffer from the condition. The family is a potentially important source of support for the person with diabetes, especially when they enter the stage of chronic disability.

Suggested aim for this session
For participants to explore the experience of diabetes within the family, and consider both positive and negative implications of this wider context.

Suggested learning objectives for this session
By the end of this session, participants should be able to:
- describe the family connections of a person with diabetes using a genogram or other written diagram
- discuss the concept of the extended family, and give examples of how the reality of family and social support for people with diabetes may differ from this ideal
- provide basic advice to a person with diabetes about the risk to their children and other relatives of developing diabetes.

Suggestions for group exercises
When you have read the story in the Box, try one or more of the following:

1. Discuss the story and genogram of Mrs S, Mr Miah, Mrs Uddin, or Mr JD, or all four. In what ways is diabetes a "family problem" in these cases? What role does the family play – and what role *should* it play – in each case? How should health professionals interact with the immediate and extended family?
2. Share your own stories of "diabetes in the family" using genograms to aid your discussions. When constructing your genogram, use different colours to delineate (a) the index case (the person you are discussing); (b) any relatives with diabetes (including long-dead ancestors), giving the age and cause of death if available; (c) the people who provide information and support to the index case.

3. Think about the patients whose stories you have discussed. What advice should you give these individuals about their own children's risk of diabetes?

Suggested assignment

Draw a genogram of a person with diabetes using similar notation to that shown for Mr Miah. Write a page about the family relationships and how they affect (a) the person's risk of diabetes and their chance of complications, and (b) the person's family support (or lack of it). When you have done this, write a paragraph about *how* the health professionals should take the family situation into account in your chosen case.

Further reading

An article for health professionals about diabetes in South Asians
Greenhalgh PM. Diabetes in British South Asians: nature, nurture and culture. *Diabetic Med* 1997;**11**:10–14.

An article for health professionals about inheritance of diabetes
Pierce M, Hayworth J, Warburton F, Keen H, Bradley C. Diabetes mellitus in the family: perceptions of offspring's risk. *Diabetic Med* 1999;**16**:431–6.

Diabetes UK website – for professionals and the public
http://www.diabetes.org.uk/

The story of Mrs S

Mrs S was diagnosed with diabetes when she was pregnant with her last child in 1985. Since then she has continued to have diabetes – tablet and diet controlled. Mrs S is very inactive, does not exercise or do housework. Her husband and daughters cook for her. They cook brown rice.

Mrs S has been very depressed since her father died. She worries a lot about everything. She blames her caesarean in 1985 for her lack of activity! She reads a lot and is quite scared of the diabetes "horror stories" she's heard from people. Mrs S is very stubborn, however, and it is hard to convince her to seek help for depression.

Mrs S loves shopping and shops for hours. She has a friend/neighbour who is diabetic. They talk to each other, usually complaining about their ailments. Her friend, however, is very active and has a very controlled diet. Mrs S doesn't go out much unless for shopping! She has many relatives in the UK. She speaks on the phone a lot but visits to relatives are not very frequent.

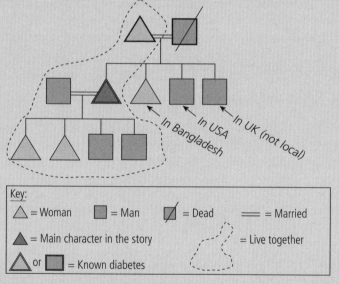

Key:

△ = Woman ■ = Man ◪ = Dead ══ = Married

▲ = Main character in the story ⌇ = Live together

△ or ■ = Known diabetes

Mrs S's family tree

What are the learning points?

The story shows how scary diabetes is for some people and how they become depressed. Also both Mrs S's parents had diabetes but none of her brothers or sisters have it yet. It could be to do with their lifestyle. Mrs S is lucky she has a supportive environment, it could be a lot worse. Stress and anxiety can be factors that affect diabetes.

Tutor's comment

As this narrator rightly points out, this woman is benefiting from family and social support. Without it, her depressing situation could be very much worse. Nevertheless, as this case illustrates, we should not assume that family support can alleviate the anguish of diabetes or replace professional help when it is needed.

The story of Mr Miah

Mr Miah, newly arrived in England, is a 26-year-old restaurant worker. At a regular health check at his GP's surgery, sugar was found in his urine sample. Mr Miah was sent for a blood test and the results showed that he was diabetic. The nurse advised him about diet control and checked his urine to test his sugar levels. I (the advocate) talked to him about buying a blood-testing machine so he could check his blood to give him a more accurate reading of his sugar levels. Mr Miah was not very shocked about his diagnosis because he said his father was diabetic, all his uncles were diabetic and he was used to hearing the word "diabetes" because most of his family had it. Mr Miah decided to buy a blood-testing machine as he said he was very young and wanted to monitor his diabetes carefully and to see if his eating habits and diet were well controlled.

Why did you choose this story?

Mr Miah was one of my first clients who was diagnosed with type 2 diabetes at 26 years old, while normally my diabetic clients are 40 years old and over.

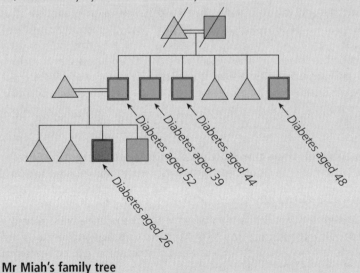

Mr Miah's family tree

Could anything have been done differently?
Because Mr Miah was newly registered and diagnosed immediately not much could have been done differently. He was diagnosed and advised at the first opportunity.

What questions or issues does this story raise?
Mr Miah could have been diabetic for some time. He mentioned feeling very unwell and tired for about 8 months.

What are the learning points?
Even though he knew about the risks of diabetes in his family he never thought of checking himself. People still don't understand the difference between "knowing about diabetes in the family" and having diabetes yourself. More health promotion work needs to be done in this area.

Tutor's comment
This narrator correctly identified an important problem in families with a high incidence of diabetes. Although the patient knew he was at high risk of diabetes, it took him a long time to get his symptoms checked out. The family and the community knew about diabetes, but the potential benefit of preventive lifestyle action (for example, exercise, weight control) and the need for prompt diagnosis and early treatment were overlooked.

The story of Mrs Uddin
Mrs Uddin is a 35-year-old Bengali woman. She is 20 weeks pregnant and already has three children. Mrs Uddin recently came to this country and was diagnosed with diabetes. She had to face many difficulties. She was missing her family in Bangladesh. Her husband works outside London and visits twice a week. She therefore stays with her in-laws. Mrs Uddin was expecting her husband to take her to the GP. She was feeling very tired. When she eventually saw the midwife she found out she was diabetic. She had to start taking insulin for which she was dependent on others. Her grandmother and father had also been diabetic. Her father had not taken care of his health and he died at the age of 50.

Learning she was insulin dependent was frightening for Mrs Uddin and caused her to become depressed. She did not understand why she had to take insulin and thought it might cause her to die like her father. Due to language barriers that existed, Mrs Uddin found it difficult to get the necessary help when she needed it. She relied on her sister-in-law to inject her with insulin, but she often had to wait for a long time for her medication as her sister-in-law was busy. Mrs Uddin had been to the hospital a few times. The linkworker and health advocate had been regularly monitoring her progress and feeding back the information to the health professionals.

Why did you choose this story?
Because of the many difficulties Mrs Uddin had to face being diagnosed with diabetes away from home.

What questions or issues does this story raise?
Through the advocates Mrs Uddin realised that not taking her insulin properly would result in detrimental effects on her unborn baby.

What are the learning points?
Mrs Uddin became much more responsible for her own health and had more help from her extended family once they had gained knowledge about the condition and how to treat it. Mrs Uddin did not previously understand diabetes and found it difficult to treat herself. After being advised by the linkworker and health advocate Mrs Uddin realised the seriousness of her condition and started making sure she took her medication regularly.

Tutor's comment
This story illustrates a number of issues common in a family with diabetes. First, there is a positive family history and a "horror story" of a relative suffering early death. Second, family members with previous experience of caring for diabetes are not around when the new case is diagnosed (in this case, because they are back in Bangladesh). Third, contrary to the popular stereotype, the support from this Asian extended family is inadequate – those who are competent to help also have their own lives to lead. Finally, there is a strong suggestion of both guilt and despair in the diabetic member: she is dependent on her relatives but also conscious of being a burden to them.

The story of Mr JD

This story is about a man of 49 who was very overweight and weighed 17 stone. He was frequently told to go on a diet and to take regular exercise – he could not do much exercise because of a foot problem – but he was convinced that because his father and grandfather had had diabetes, he would have it as well anyway. He didn't select the kinds of foods he ate and he smoked excessively. He became insulin dependent and was admitted to hospital suffering strokes.

Mr JD's father had died of a stroke, as well as his grandfather. His wife tries to look after him; he does not work and stays home. It is frustrating for his wife. Mr JD has regular strokes and heart attacks, at least three times a year. In the past it used to be four or five times. He has lost 2 stone now but still smokes.

Why did you choose this story?

This is a story of hereditary diabetes and the man is an obese person who smokes heavily.

Could anything have been done differently?

Mr JD should check his feet every day and report any signs of discomfort. A regular routine should be followed, such as washing feet, exercising daily, and most importantly discontinuing smoking because it makes the blood flow to the feet worse.

What questions or issues does this story raise?

It shows the effects that an unhealthy diet and no exercise can produce. Careless concern for the feet can make the diabetes situation worse. Also a negative attitude does not help the situation in any way.

What are the learning points?

A daily routine of looking after, checking, and caring for the feet should be followed. The fact that Mr JD is at home all the time, not adopting any form of exercise and following an unhealthy diet, is putting stress on him and his wife. Mr JD should be regularly escorted to his diabetes clinic appointments and maybe should stay in hospital for a few days to help him adopt a new lifestyle and routine.

Tutor's comment

This narrator was clearly frustrated by Mr JD's fatalistic attitude and self neglect, which contrasts markedly with that of Mr Miah, who was keen to take good care of himself once diagnosed. The question of whether poor outcomes of diabetes in certain families are due to "nature" or "nurture" is debated, but this patient probably learnt his negative attitudes and behaviour within the family. The narrator correctly identifies the need for intensive education and perhaps supervised clinic visits – though hospital admission is unlikely to help in the long term.

Unit 4
Check-ups and visits to the doctor

Background

The cornerstone of good diabetes management is said to be the "three Rs" – registration, recall, and regular review – that is, every person with diabetes should be called up for regular check-ups, even when they don't feel ill. At these check-up visits, the patient should be offered a review of their diabetes control, a physical check for the early, treatable stages of complications (such as high blood pressure, eye problems or foot problems), and time to discuss their concerns about diabetes. The reality is often very different. Diabetic clinics can be busy, impersonal, and confusing, especially for the patient who speaks little English. They may have no idea what tests are being done or why, and their own concerns and priorities may be overlooked. Small wonder, then, that non-attendance rates at diabetic clinics are typically around 25%.

Suggested aim for this session

For participants to explore the meaning of check-ups and other clinic visits to people with diabetes, the hopes and fears associated with these, and the barriers to attendance.

Suggested learning objectives for this session

By the end of this session, participants should be able to:

- describe examples of different patient perspectives on the purpose of routine clinic visits
- explain in broad terms the purpose of routine diabetes surveillance to patients and their relatives
- empathise with a patient who has concerns about a visit to a clinic or hospital
- identify barriers to clinic attendance in particular patients and suggest ways of overcoming these
- support patients or clients who wish to book unscheduled visits to health professionals to discuss concerns about their diabetes.

Suggestions for group exercises

When you have read the stories for this unit, try one or more of the following:

1. Discuss the stories in this unit of Mr Alom, Mr Miah, Mrs Khanoum, and Mrs SB. What do these stories tell us about the purpose and priority of check-ups

and clinic visits from the perspective of the patient? What measures should be in place to make sure that all these patients receive the best care?

2. Share stories in your group about people who have had problems with clinic visits. Include examples from your own experience of:
   - people who have failed to attend for blood tests or check-ups
   - people who have found the clinic experience frustrating or frightening
   - people who received tests or treatments they didn't expect or didn't understand
   - people who conceal aspects of their condition from health professionals
   - people who have overcome these or similar difficulties.

Use these stories as the basis for a multidisciplinary workshop in which you improve the design of the service you currently offer.

Suggested assignment

Write two pages about how you might improve a diabetic clinic or other service for people with diabetes to make it more "user friendly". Base your account on at least one story discussed in your group. You should include at least three major suggestions for improvement and give details of *how* things should change.

Further reading

An article for health professionals about "lost to follow-up" patients
Griffin SJ. Lost to follow-up: the problem of defaulters from diabetes clinics. *Diabetic Med* 1998;**15** Suppl 3: S14–24.

A guide for patients on what to expect at check-ups
What diabetes care to expect. This booklet provides information on what diabetes care you should expect from the NHS, your diabetes care team, and if you are ill and in hospital. Available free from Diabetes UK (see p. 8 for details).

Diabetes UK website – for professionals and the public
http://www.diabetes.org.uk/

The story of Mr Alom

Mr Alom is a 38-year-old man. He was not taking any medication for his diabetes, it was controlled by diet. Mr Alom started complaining about feeling thirsty, passing urine frequently etc. Mr Alom was worried about his diabetes and he wanted a blood test. He was given a blood test form at his GP's.

Why did you choose this story?
To show that some patients are responsible for their diabetes.

What are the learning points?
This patient knew his symptoms were getting worse.

Tutor's comment

This short account demonstrates that routine check-up visits are designed to supplement, not replace, the patient's own surveillance of their diabetes. This patient knew he was deteriorating and also knew that he needed a blood test. Less assertive patients may need prompting to respond to their symptoms by booking an appointment; others may need practical help to do this.

The story of Mr Miah

Mr Miah is a 63-year-old man. For 3 months he has been coming to see the nurse for asthma checks. The nurse checked his blood sugar to see if Mr Miah might be diabetic and it tested at 5·3. She sent him for a further blood test (glucose tolerance test or GTT). Mr Miah did not go three times. We were still not sure about Mr Miah as his sugar levels were always around 5·3 to 5·4 (which is borderline). Finally, Mr Miah admitted why he didn't go for a GTT. He is scared of having blood taken. He believes he doesn't have enough blood.

The nurse was understanding and explained why it was necessary for him to have a GTT. Mr Miah still looked unsure and I believe he will still not go if referred for GTT. The outcome was to see Mr Miah every month so the nurse could check him with a finger prick blood test and monitor him regularly as he is borderline.

Why did you choose this story?
It shows a case of a man who never goes for blood tests to find out if he is diabetic.

Could anything have been done differently?
I think nothing could have been done differently because Mr Miah is scared of having blood tests and the only way to help him understand is by listening to him and monitoring him.

What questions or issues does this story raise?
- Do many people miss blood tests because they are scared?
- Does everybody understand about GTT?

What are the learning points?
- Some patients have fears
- Some patients do not understand why GTT is important.

Tutor's comment
See the next story.

The story of Mrs Khanoum
Mrs Khanoum is a 45-year-old housewife and mother who speaks no English. Diagnosed with diabetes, Mrs Khanoum was given an appointment time by her GP for a check-up. Two months later when her check-up appointment date arrived, she did not attend. The professionals were confused as to why Mrs Khanoum did not attend, given the importance of monitoring diabetes and regular check-ups. Mrs Khanoum took her appointment card from her GP for her check-up. She realised later that the appointment was for 9.30 am, a time when she takes her children to school. She could not speak English to explain that this time was inconvenient.

Mrs Khanoum went back to the GP complaining of worsening symptoms, that is, dizzy spells. On this occasion a Bengali health advocate was available to provide language support and to find out why Mrs Khanoum did not attend her last appointment.

Why did you choose this story?
The story highlights a reason why clients do not go to their health clinic for check-ups.

Could anything have been done differently?
A health advocate should have been available from the beginning to explain to Mrs Kahnoum why check-ups are important and to find out what the barriers were to her attending her check-up.

What questions or issues does this story raise?
- Language support required for some Bengali clients
- Full explanation of importance of check-ups needs to be given
- Check appointment times, particularly for mothers: they should not be at school dropping off and picking up times.

What are the learning points?

Cultural sensitivity for specific community groups needs to be taken into account and relevant health promotion and awareness is required.

Tutor's comment

This story, and the previous story of Mr Miah, reflect the frustration many of us have felt when we put effort into fixing tests or consultations for patients who then fail to turn up. But they usually have their reasons, and both narrators have found out exactly why their patients didn't attend. One patient believed that the test would be bad for him (he'd lose too much blood), and the other had a simple, practical, and important reason why she could not make the time given. Furthermore, neither of them understood the purpose of the visit nor its importance for their health.

The story of Mrs SB

This is about Mrs SB, a 60-year-old housewife who could not speak English and did not understand or care about her condition of diabetes. When she did realise the importance and consequences of her condition she blamed the health professionals at her GP's surgery for not looking after her. She is now in a wheelchair and has lost her eyesight and has to go for kidney dialysis. Mrs SB ignored her medication and the tablets given to her and now she is more aware and cautious.

The doctor had no idea that Mrs SB had not followed the medication and when he phoned her she lied frequently and told the doctor she was fine. Therefore, the doctor had no responsibility for the consequences. Now Mrs SB is a lot more aware and cautious and disciplined. She has her niece to look after her and is using insulin because her sugars are high. She takes her niece to interpret at appointments and has regular check-ups. Mrs SB is also careful with her diet and exercises her feet.

Why did you choose this story?

To identify the educational needs of health professionals in relation to Bangladeshi culture.

Could anything have been done differently?

Mrs SB is now well aware that if things had been followed differently the extent of her present condition would have been lessened. However, she was not aware of the consequences and treated the diabetes less severely. She could have contacted her family if she had doubts or did not understand.

What questions or issues does this story raise?
It raises the issue that health professionals should be more aware of the lack of knowledge and experiences that Bangladeshi people have regarding diabetes. If in doubt that the patient does not understand, and on behalf of the health professionals, the patient's family should be contacted.

What are the learning points?
- A diabetes awareness day for Bangladeshi people or communities could be held to make them more aware of the consequences of diabetes.
- Eyes and feet, in particular, are parts of the body which are not checked regularly and should be paid more attention.
- Communication difficulties between health professionals and Bangladeshi patients should also be identified. A survey should be conducted or statistical data compiled to show the effects of poor health outcomes of lack of diabetes care.

Tutor's comment
This tragic story reminds us that some patients, especially those from certain ethnic groups, may be tempted to tell health professionals what they think they want to hear. If we are to prevent people like Mrs SB from the devastating complication of diabetes, we must acknowledge and overcome problems such as denial, profound lack of understanding, and the desire to please the doctor or nurse.

Unit 5
Medication

Background

Diabetes may be treated with lifestyle measures alone (see Unit 6) or with tablets or insulin, but there is no cure, and patients need to continue medication for the rest of their lives. Additional problems like high blood pressure or cholesterol are common, and may also require drug treatment. Furthermore, the natural tendency of type 2 diabetes is to get steadily worse with time, which means that even if patients work hard at controlling their diabetes, they will probably need to take more and more drugs as they get older.

Many patients take over-the-counter remedies (such as vitamins and tonics) and alternative therapies (such as herbs) for their diabetes. In traditional societies, most illness occurs as acute episodes (for example, diarrhoeal disease, malaria), and medication, if effective at all, generally cures the problem quickly. People coming from such societies may have trouble understanding the need for long-term medication that does not cure. Fear of taking insulin in some Asian patients is sometimes compounded by an incorrect belief that all insulin is derived from beef.

Suggested aim for this session

For participants to explore the ideas, concerns, expectations, and experiences of patients with respect to medication for diabetes.

Suggested learning objectives for this session

By the end of this session, participants should be able to:
- give a basic account of the methods of treating diabetes (diet alone, tablets, insulin) and the expected changes to medication as the disease progresses
- describe the range of perceptions held by patients about tablets and insulin
- identify potential barriers to compliance with medication and suggest ways of overcoming these.

Suggestions for group exercises

Read the stories in the Box and then try one or more of the following:

1. Discuss the different stories in this unit, and also the other stories about medication on pp. 44–5, 50, 56, and 61. Make a list of all the issues they raise.
2. Share stories within your group about patients' attitudes towards medication and problems that have arisen. If anyone in your group takes regular

medication themselves, or has to administer it to a relative, hear their story too.

3. Design a prompt chart to be used by a doctor, nurse, pharmacist or advocate when explaining to a patient that they need to start insulin. You do not need to address the clinical aspects (such as how much to take, when, and how). Instead, focus on the barriers to effective medication we have considered here and think of ways to overcome them.

Suggested assignment

Imagine you have been asked by a group of doctors to give them a brief summary of how cultural issues might affect their patients' adherence to medication (you can choose tablets, insulin, or both). Make a list of at least five key points and give examples of real or imaginary patients that illustrate each point. For each point, suggest ways in which the doctors could change their practice to improve adherence.

Further reading

A guide to diabetes medication for health professionals

MacKinnon M. *Providing diabetes care in general practice: a practical guide for the primary health care team*, 4th edition. London: Class Publishing, 2002. See ch. 8, "Drug and insulin therapy", pp. 97–116.

An article for health professionals about compliance with medication

Lutfey KE, Wishner WJ. Beyond "compliance" is "adherence". Improving the prospect of diabetes care. *Diabetes Care* 1999;**22**:635–9.

A guide to diabetes medication for patients

Booklets on both tablets and insulin are available free from Diabetes UK (see pp. 8 for details).

Diabetes UK website – for professionals and the public

http://www.diabetes.org.uk/

The story of Mrs Begum

Mrs Begum came to the clinic for her diabetes check. A blood test showed that her sugars were very high. The nurse advised Mrs Begum that in the future she might need to go on insulin. Mrs Begum was not prepared to take injections. She was scared of needles. The nurse was also worried about her patient's diabetic control. Mrs Begum decided to join a fitness class and to watch her diet more carefully.

Why did you choose this story?
It was an interesting example.

What questions or issues does this story raise?
Mrs Begum would do anything to avoid insulin injections.

What are the learning points?
Many patients have a great fear of needles.

The story of Mrs J

Mrs J is a woman of 45 who is afraid to take conventional medication for her diabetes. She was prescribed medication for two months by her doctor but she doesn't take it, she throws it away. She is afraid of side effects like heart attacks and strokes.

Why did you choose this story?
It is a story about a woman who thought conventional medication was not good for her.

Could anything have been done differently?
The woman could have been provided with more information and encouraged to talk to different people who have taken the same medication.

What questions or issues does this story raise?
This person did not believe in medication and is not willing to take it as she doesn't believe in conventional medication.

What are the learning points?
Although diet and exercise are also vital, this woman must be encouraged further to take the medication. This will help build up her trust in conventional medication.

Tutor's comment
We all know that patients often do not take their medication as directed. These two stories show that patients generally have good reasons for what we call "non-compliance". The

narrators have identified some important measures that may help improve compliance: exploring concerns, explaining how drugs work and why they are needed, and arranging for the patient to talk to someone with experience of the same drug. However, the first story also demonstrates that "non-compliance" can have positive outcomes – Mrs Begum was so keen to avoid insulin that she made some major (and successful) lifestyle changes.

The story of Mrs A

Mrs A was on holiday in the USA. She was on high doses of insulin. When she was about to use her insulin she found she only had a little left and she panicked. She went to the chemist but couldn't get insulin without a doctor's prescription. She asked if she could buy it but was refused. Mrs A was upset in case she didn't find a doctor and the chemist was not helpful in giving her information on what to do next. Finally, she started to exercise more and eat less.

Could anything have been done differently?
The woman should have taken out travel insurance.

What questions or issues does this story raise?
Diabetes is a serious illness and can make you feel very unwell and not able to enjoy a holiday at the same time.

What are the learning points?
Diabetic patients should be careful and get much more information on diabetes before they travel.

The taxi story

Two distant relatives were diabetes sufferers. One was about 60 years old living in Newham, the other a child of 10 living in Hackney. On one occasion (it was a weekend), when the mother of the 10-year-old child realised that her daughter's insulin had run out and the child was not feeling well, the mother phoned her older relative for advice on what to do in such a situation. On hearing this, the 60-year-old woman offered her own medication (tablets) and confidently explained that she was suffering from the same illness. She found her medication to be very effective. The mother of the 10-year-old gladly agreed to the proposal. Later it was decided that the old lady would take her medication by mini cab to Hackney.

While the two women were on the phone the daughter of the older woman, who worked for a health care trust, came in and overheard the conversation. When she realised what was going on, she intervened and tried to explain the danger of medicine sharing, but with no success at all. The old woman left for Hackney to deliver her tablets. Her daughter then chased her in another cab. Fortunately both arrived in Hackney at the same time. The older woman's daughter was able to stop the younger girl taking the tablets by saying she would get an emergency supply of insulin from the local hospital. Finally, they all went to the hospital and got insulin to cover the weekend.

This story was related in our group by a member who had also been involved in the Community Pharmacy Project (Syed Shahriar, Project Evaluation, Social Action for Health, 2000)

Tutor's comment

Insulin is literally essential for life, but there are many different forms of insulin and pharmacists are rightly reluctant to replenish supplies without clear instructions from a doctor. Tablets are usually no help for a person who is dependent on insulin, and may be dangerous. Information on how to take medication should be given repeatedly and should include instructions on what to do if the medication runs out.

Unit 6
Supporting positive lifestyle choices

Background

The management of diabetes requires the patient to adopt a healthy lifestyle – in particular, to give up smoking, to reduce body weight if overweight, to take a diet high in complex carbohydrates (such as brown rice) and low in fat (such as ghee), and to take strenuous exercise for at least half an hour on most days. The active involvement of the patient in his or her own care is therefore crucial to the success of any management plan. But as anyone who has tried to give up smoking, change their diet or increase their exercise level knows, these aspects of our lives are not easy to change. Resistance to change can occur on a practical, psychological, and cultural level.

Suggested aim for this session

For participants to explore the lived experience of diabetes with particular reference to healthy lifestyle choices.

Suggested learning objectives for this session

By the end of this session, participants should be able to:

- give a basic account of the lifestyle considered best for people with diabetes (see "Background" above and "Further reading" below)
- give examples of barriers to positive lifestyle choices in patients with diabetes and suggest ways to overcome these for particular patients
- support individual patients, and groups of people with diabetes, in learning more about positive lifestyle choices (for example, through exercise programmes or healthy eating classes).

Suggestions for group exercises

When you have read the stories on pp. 35–40, try one or more of the following:

1. Discuss your own smoking, eating, and exercise habits within your group. How easy would you find it to stop smoking, lose weight, follow a "diabetic diet", or exercise for half an hour or more every day? What would be the main barriers – "addiction", preference, religious or cultural restrictions, cost, or convenience? How might you overcome each of those?

2. Plan (and, if possible, deliver) a "taster" educational session on some aspect of lifestyle change for a group of patients with diabetes. This could be:
   - a cookery demonstration (what would you cook?)
   - an exercise class designed for a traditionally less active group (for example, older south Asian women)
   - a support group for smoking cessation or weight control.

Suggested assignment

Work on a one-to-one basis with an individual client and support them through a lifestyle change. Make careful notes on their efforts and the problems they encounter. If they are unsuccessful, try to discover what went wrong. Write an account of (a) what went well, and why you think it did; (b) what went less well, and what you or the patient might do differently next time.

Further reading

Books and articles on lifestyle for health professionals
Lancaster T, Stead L, Silagy C, Sowden A. Effectiveness of interventions to help people stop smoking: findings from the Cochrane Library. *BMJ* 2000;**321**:355–8.
Macaulay D. *Benefits and hazards of sport and exercise.* London: BMJ Publications, 1999.

Leaflets and books on lifestyle issues for people with diabetes
Several leaflets on lifestyle available free from Diabetes UK (see p. 8 for details), and downloadable from the website below.
Thomas M, Greene LW. *The unofficial guide to living with diabetes (MacMillan Lifestyles Guide).* New York: Hungry Minds, 1999.

Diabetes UK website – for professionals and the public
Information on exercise: http://www.diabetes.org.uk/manage/physical/splash.htm
Information on eating: http://www.diabetes.org.uk/manage/eatwell/eatwell.htm

Alternative Diabetes website – intended mainly for the public
This website has many ideas about living with diabetes and has a non-medical focus on lifestyle without being anti-medicine.
http://www.alternativediabetes.com

The story of Mrs Miah

Mrs Miah, a 60-year-old housewife, was overweight, did little exercise, and her main diet consisted of the rich foods (that is, high in fat), with little fruit or vegetables, of the traditional housewife. At the age of 60 Mrs Miah was diagnosed as having diabetes by her GP and was advised she could control it through diet and improvement of lifestyle. Mrs Miah did not monitor her diabetes or improve her lifestyle. As a result 6 months later her GP advised her that she needed to go on insulin.

Mrs Miah knew little about diabetes; what little she did know were "horror stories" (namely, the removal of limbs). She did not understand the importance of monitoring and improving her lifestyle to prevent her condition getting worse and thought ignoring it would help. Ignoring the condition, not improving her diet or leading a more active lifestyle over a 6 month period meant Mrs Miah was now insulin dependent and the options available to her before were now closed.

Mrs Miah now regularly attends swimming classes and the gym every week. She also regularly attends a support group. It's a shame she never accessed these activities before she learnt she had to start taking insulin.

Why did you choose this story?

To show lack of awareness about monitoring and looking after your diabetes (that is, better diet and lifestyle) can make the condition worse. Ignoring the condition will not make it go away.

Could anything have been done differently?

Mrs Miah should have been given information about support groups for patients with diabetes, making her more willing to accept her condition and deal with it, through learning about monitoring and preventing diabetes getting worse.

What questions or issues does this story raise?

Promotion of awareness helps alleviate the shock of knowing you have diabetes and helps you to deal with the condition more effectively. Support groups could prevent feelings of isolation and can be very educational.

What are the learning points?

Prevention is better than cure. It is cheaper in the long run and causes less distress to the patient concerned, particularly in this case study where the patient's condition was worsened due to lack of awareness, resulting in not prioritising her health during the first 6 months of diagnosis.

Tutor's comment

The narrator is probably right that the lack of self-care and positive lifestyle choices in the early months of this patient's diabetes contributed to the need for insulin at an early stage. However, lifestyle measures may or may not have prevented the need for insulin altogether. This story suggests that patients may enter a phase of hopelessness and self-neglect soon after the diagnosis is made, and that a potential way to prevent this and provide essential education on *how* to change lifestyle is social support through a diabetes group – discussed in some of the other stories in this unit.

The story of Mrs Khatun

Mrs Khatun is a 45-year-old housewife. She was diagnosed as having diabetes 5 years ago. She was advised by her GP to eat less oily food and more fruit and vegetables. Mrs Khatun had cooked and prepared food with a high oil and spice content for her family for years and continued to do so. She did not think curries could be made or taste nice with less oil and spice. Mrs Khatun took her diabetes medication but did not know how to prepare food with less oil and spices, hence she continued cooking in the same way. Through her neighbour, she heard about health sessions for women who wanted to improve their lifestyles but didn't know how. During these sessions women discussed their experiences, were given health literature and cooking demonstrations. Mrs Khatun attended the sessions regularly at her local community centre.

What questions or issues does this story raise?

Much health promotion literature dictates that people should improve their lifestyle but does not mention how. Not everyone can read/write Bengali so they throw the literature away. Many diabetics would improve their diet if they knew how to do it.

What are the learning points?

Diabetics could improve their lifestyle and diet through a holistic approach including health sessions, cooking demonstrations, and literature, rather than one being used in isolation.

The story of AB

A previously healthy 10-year-old boy, AB, discovered a few months ago that he had diabetes. He lost a lot of weight, felt thirsty, frequently went to the loo and his lips were very dry. His Mum, who cares for him – his father is not around as they are divorced – took him to the hospital and his blood sugar was tested. It was very high and the doctors said he should go on a careful diet (as well as insulin). So his Mum always gives him boiled food and now he is fed up and frustrated and he feels tired most of the time. His Mum is very worried and so are the doctors at his lack of enthusiasm and lack of concentration and interest in his studies. He knows how to take his insulin himself. His Mum taught him. Sometimes, AB sneaks down chocolates and his blood sugars get very high and he needs to stay in hospital and his insulin dose is increased. But he is scared about insulin and blood testing in hospitals. He doesn't want to go but his Mum forces him.

Could anything have been done differently?
The boy's mother should not have been so strict with his diet by limiting it to only boiled vegetables. She should vary the diet and adapt recipes with, for example, lower oil content, less salt and sugar which is always found in large amounts in Asian Bangladeshi foods.

What questions or issues does this story raise?
It is a very emotional upheaval for a 10-year-old boy to cope with diabetes and a big responsibility for a young person going to start secondary school soon. The mother feels guilty and occasionally when her other son eats chocolate she allows AB to have it as well.

What are the learning points?
The diet, most of all, should be varied. Although the boy is not overweight, he should exercise regularly to improve his well-being and raise his energy levels so that his studies, which are very important, improve. If he follows a regular exercise programme and controls his diet, it will give him an advantage when he is elderly. It will also become enjoyable to a young, growing boy.

Tutor's comment
The barrier to healthy and palatable food choices in both these cases was simple ignorance. As the first narrator suggests, there's nothing like a practical demonstration when it comes to cooking!

The story of Mrs A

Mrs A, a 35-year-old diet controlled diabetic woman, has to monitor her blood sugars at home. Her blood goes very high every night and sometimes at lunch time. The doctor said, if it goes on like this, she may need insulin. Talking to Mrs A I found out that her husband comes home late every night and Mrs A eats at that time with him. Her diet is not very good. She eats one whole honey mango every night. After eating she checks her blood and goes to bed. Whenever she comes to clinic she doesn't eat breakfast in case her sugar levels go too high.

Mrs A was shocked and worried about her high sugars. She reported that she does not take sugary food and no sugar in her tea. She felt confused and wanted more advice on diet. Mrs A needed to change her eating timetable and also to check her blood sugar level after two hours of intake. She should cut down her mango as mango is a sugary fruit. She agreed to follow the prescribed diet to avoid going on insulin.

Why did you choose this story?
This is a common scenario.

Could anything have been done differently?
More encouragement and reminders about following the prescribed diet. Monitor diet and make a food in-take timetable before putting people with high sugars on insulin.

What questions or issues does this story raise?
Patients may be eating the wrong foods at the wrong times. Sometimes patients misinterpret or misunderstand what is said.

What are the learning points?
Make sure the patient understands what is said. Communication is an important factor. It is important to follow dietary instructions and a regular timetable. More resources are needed to help make patients aware of their health needs.

Tutor's comment

This story illustrates that even patients who are making a serious effort to eat the right foods may unwittingly be following a poor diet. A detailed account of what is eaten, and when, will help to identify avoidable pitfalls. This story also illustrates the feelings of guilt and frustration that patients experience when their personal efforts do not produce results.

Another of our group members told a similar story, and concluded that health professionals should visit patients' houses, look in their cupboards and observe mealtimes to find out what is actually being cooked and how; and who eats the food, when, and in what quantities.

The story of Mrs LM

Mrs LM, aged 60, was diagnosed with diabetes. She is an elderly woman who smokes. She has accepted the diabetes as a matter of growing old gracefully. She was given literature about exercise which she did not read. Exercise was not part of her daily routine, she did not prioritise it as something important, and felt it would not help her situation.

Mrs LM felt she was old anyway and that exercise could not in any way help to enhance her life or relieve her condition. Then she attended "Befriending Health Sessions" in a local community centre. These were culturally sensitive and for women only, where the importance of exercise and diet for diabetics was highlighted. Discussions also took place which were much more effective than literature – which people do not always read. Literature combined with health sessions seem to work better, you can't have the one without the other.

Mrs LM now attends swimming classes for women only at a local community centre. She does not have to wear a swimming costume but can wear her shalwar kameez.

Why did you choose this story?

To highlight the lack of awareness and promotion of exercise linked to diabetes and how it can help relieve the condition. To show how the issues of cultural barriers can prevent people from attending exercise classes.

Could anything have been done differently?

Mrs LM was only given leaflets about exercise which she did not read. She should have been referred to community health sessions straight away where she would have access to culturally sensitive exercise.

What questions or issues does this story raise?

Many women cannot access exercise classes for a number of reasons: sessions are mixed, or changing and shower rooms are communal or the clothes they wear are awkward.

What are the learning points?

More effective health promotion and awareness around exercise is needed, stressing its importance. More culturally sensitive exercise classes are needed.

Tutor's comment

This story again demonstrates the value of "show" rather than "tell" in relation to healthy lifestyle choices, and of the social group in prompting and supporting lifestyle changes. It also shows the importance of good communication and liaison between health professionals and voluntary and community initiatives. The doctor or nurse who merely gave the patient an unintelligible leaflet would surely have referred directly to the Befriending Health Sessions if he or she had known about it.

The story of Mr Ahmed

Mr Ahmed was 56 years old and an insulin dependent diabetic. He used to be quite active and an outgoing person. He had one bad habit, he used to smoke a lot. The doctor told him to give up smoking but he did not take it seriously. His daughter used to hide his cigarettes; generally he did not mind about it but sometimes he got very desperate and got very angry about getting the cigarettes.

Mr Ahmed used to say some people died of heart attacks and lung cancer but they never smoked. He used to say, "My sugar level is not going high so I am alright. I will die when my time is up and nobody can change that". The outcome, however, was very sad. Mr Ahmed had two heart attacks. After that he was a very different person. He went to Mecca for Haj. After that he used to spend most of his time praying. Then he had a third heart attack and died.

Why did you choose this story?

The story is meaningful about lifestyle and has a sad ending.

Could anything have been done differently?

Mr Ahmed should have had more counselling on the effects of smoking. He should have met more people who suffer from the same problems and have been given information leaflets on the effects of smoking.

What questions or issues does this story raise?

Mr Ahmed was addicted to cigarettes, he could not give up, his will power was not strong enough and he turned to religion for solace.

What are the learning points?

- The doctor's advice should not be taken lightly: smoking causes more harm to people with diabetes.
- Television plays a big part in everybody's lives. The government should make a series of programmes on health issues to show us.

Tutor's comment

Every smoker has a story about someone who smoked heavily and lived to 99 – but people who succumb to the effects of their smoking may not live to tell the tale! As in this tragic story, smoking is a serious addiction and its impact on patients with diabetes is often devastating. The narrator rightly states that assistance with smoking cessation can be provided through individual counselling, "doctor's orders", and via the mass media. In addition, drugs and patches can be prescribed by a doctor – see "Further reading" for details.

Unit 7
Loneliness and lack of support

Background
When we ran our first Sharing Stories group, we were struck by the number of stories about people with diabetes who lacked social support and who encountered more than their share of problems with lifestyle, medication, clinic attendance, and diabetic complications. We came to the conclusion that the support of the family and the community is an essential prerequisite for good quality of life and health outcomes in diabetes.

Suggested aim for this session
For participants to explore the impact of poor social support in people with diabetes, and consider ways of overcoming this problem.

Suggested learning objectives for this session
By the end of this session, participants should be able to:
- give an account of the lived experience of diabetes in a person with little social support
- describe the potential adverse outcomes of the cycle of ignorance, fear, hopelessness, and self-neglect that often accompanies this lack of support
- identify patients who have, or are at risk of, these problems and suggest measures to address them for particular individuals.

Suggestions for group exercises
When you have read the stories in this unit, and also the story of Mrs Begum on p. 4, try one or more of the following:

1. Discuss these stories, and share any stories on similar themes from within your group. How common are your examples? Of course, there are no easy answers to these complex problems, but think about *why* social isolation appears to have such a dramatic impact on diabetes in particular.
2. Take a patient with complex needs and social isolation. List systematically all their different problems. Now, in a multidisciplinary group, plan an "ideal" package of care for that patient. Include the patient's friends and relatives if there are any, and lay and voluntary groups. When you have planned the "ideal" package, consider barriers to achieving this in practice and try to

construct a compromise that takes account of competing demands on everyone's time and stress levels.

Suggested assignment

Write up the second exercise above as an essay with the following subheadings:
- The story from the patient's perspective
- The patient's needs – including health care, social care, and other
- The proposed care package
- The staff needed to deliver that package: who will do what?
- A conclusion

Further reading

Articles for health professionals about social support and diabetes

Brown SA, Hanis CL. A community-based, culturally sensitive education and group-support intervention for Mexican Americans with NIDDM: a pilot study of efficacy. *Diabetes Educator* 1995;**21**:203–10.

Gilden JL, Hendryx MS, Clar S, Casia C, Singh SP. Diabetes support groups improve health care of older diabetic patients. *J Am Geriatr Soci* 1992;**40**:147–50.

The story of Mrs P

Mrs P is a 47-year-old widow. She has been suffering from diabetes for 5 years, since just after her husband died. She finds it hard to cope with her diet. She feels dizzy most of the time and weak. Sometimes she feels "hypo". Her diet is not very well controlled. She felt that she was doing well but it still wasn't that good. It worries her why that is happening. She misses her husband and feels lonely most of the time. She doesn't go out and about or mix with other people. Mrs P is depressed. She does not know the facts about diabetes. She needs to go out and mix with other people who have diabetes and she needs an exercise class. Mrs P's major worry is that she's feeling lonely and missing her partner. She really needs help to talk to someone and get referred to a diabetes adviser, and to have regular check-ups.

Why did you choose this story?

Mrs P is a widow living with her son and daughter-in-law and not coping well with her diet.

Could anything have been done differently?

Mrs P needs to see a dietician for advice on food and a low sugar diet. She needs to talk to someone who can reassure her.

What questions or issues does this story raise?

Mrs P didn't know why her sugar levels go up and down. Because she feels "hypo" at times she thinks her sugar is not controlled. She really needs good advice on diet.

The story of Mrs Begum

Mrs Begum, aged 54, was diagnosed with diabetes and arthritis. She is a widow and has two daughters. Her grandmother also had diabetes. In her first pregnancy, Mrs Begum was diagnosed as a diabetic patient and her husband used to take care of her health. After her husband's death it was a great shock to her and she could not continue her insulin properly and was unable to monitor her blood tests. Eventually she became "hypo". She could not believe she was suffering from "hypos" and thought it was her arthritis. As she could not recognise the symptoms she went to her GP who arranged for her to see the district nurse. At present, the district nurse visits Mrs Begum regularly because she is unable to move about as a result of her severe arthritis and she found it difficult to keep up her appointments at the diabetic clinic.

Why did you choose this story?

Mrs Begum is very lonely and depressed and has no knowledge of how to control her diabetes.

Could anything have been done differently?
The district nurse and health advocate are teaching Mrs Begum how to use insulin and to do her blood tests. They are working closely with her.

What questions or issues does this story raise?
Although she is being given all the instructions Mrs Begum is still reluctant to do her injections and blood tests by herself.

What are the learning points?
With the help of the district nurse and health advocate Mrs Begum is now fully aware of the diabetic symptoms and understands the reasons for taking insulin and doing blood tests. Eventually, Mrs Begum will be able to take responsibility for herself.

Tutor's comment
See the next story.

The story of Mrs G

Just after her husband died, Mrs G fell ill due to a lack of proper nutrition, and shortly afterwards she was diagnosed as having diabetes. Mrs G never really came to terms with or understood her diabetes. She used to miss her insulin injections deliberately, and then she was scared of the consequences and made up for it by not eating. This was a substitute for not lowering her blood sugar levels properly. The pattern continued throughout her period of illness and it is believed to be the cause of her death. Mrs G died in hospital just as it was recognised that she was not looking after herself properly. Mrs G's family and friends felt partly responsible for her death because they were so busy and involved in their own lives they did not realise that being left alone in the house all day would encourage Mrs G's deterioration. They are full of regrets and deep disappointment.

Why did you choose this story?
The patient was a good friend of my family's for 17 years.

Could anything have been done differently?
Mrs G could have done more exercise. She used to sit inside the house all day, miserable or sleeping. Maybe a "personal trainer", or a friend and herself could have taken short walks, jogs or whatever form of exercise she enjoyed. Also Mrs G could have been better educated to know how to look after herself with diabetes.

What questions or issues does this story raise?

Can a middle-aged woman take on the responsibility of looking after herself? The doctor should have done checks (for example, blood testing) to confirm that she was as good as she said. Maybe she also needed someone to look after and support her more.

What are the learning points?

Every newly diagnosed diabetic should be given a programme of education and people should be helped to learn the principles of monitoring and control of their lifestyle to manage diabetes. Meeting other diabetics and having the chance to discuss problems may also help.

Tutor's comment

This story, and the two previous stories in this unit, illustrate the cycle of ignorance, fear, hopelessness, and self-neglect that often accompanies a lack of the social support that most people with diabetes are able to draw on to some extent. All three patients probably had depression as well as diabetes and other physical problems. It is interesting that the three narrators all came independently to similar conclusions: that patients like these need (a) more intensive input from health professionals, including education, close monitoring of their physical condition, and counselling; and (b) the opportunity to meet and share experiences with other people with diabetes.

Unit 8
Communicating across cultures

Background
It is well known that cultural differences between health professionals and patients can lead to failures in communication and unintended poor outcomes. There is much talk of "cultural sensitivity" and "cultural competence" in health care, but the challenge is to move beyond political correctness and make a real difference to outcome. The key to this task is improved understanding by "living through" rather than simply "knowing about" the experience of diabetes in different cultural settings.

Suggested aim for this session
For participants to explore the impact of language, cultural, and ethnic issues as they impact on diabetes care.

Suggested learning objectives for this session
By the end of this session, participants should be able to:
- describe the lived experience of diabetes from the perspective of someone from a different cultural background than the health professional treating them
- play the role of "cultural broker", explaining terms and customs that each side may be unfamiliar with
- identify and overcome specific barriers to effective communication between patients with diabetes and health professionals.

Suggestions for group exercises
When you have read the stories in this unit, try one or more of the following:

1. Discuss the stories of Mrs K, Mr I, and Mrs M. You could also look briefly at those on pp. 16, 24, 39, 40, 56, 57, 62, and 63, which touch on the difficulties of cross-cultural communication. Are there any clear and generalisable messages for dealing with patients from different cultures?
2. Share stories of your own experience with cultural (in)competence. Are the main problems due to ignorance, racism, practicalities (such as language), or something else? Take a single case and discuss in detail how these problems might be overcome.

3. Most of us can recall a story about a health professional who could benefit from cultural awareness training. In a multidisciplinary (and preferably multiethnic) group, plan a one-day programme of cultural awareness designed for the needs of a health professional starting right at the beginning in this field of study.

Suggested assignment

Write up a story you have shared or heard in the second exercise above. Include the following subheadings:

- The story from the patient's point of view
- The story from the health professional's point of view
- A list of the main communication problems
- A conclusion about what could be done differently to improve things next time

Further reading

A basic guide to diabetes care across cultures for health professionals

MacKinnon M. *Providing diabetes care in general practice: a practical guide for the primary health care team*, 4th edition. London: Class Publishing, 2002. See ch. 12, "Aspects of culture relating to diabetes care", pp. 157–72.

Books and articles about cross-cultural health care for professionals

Airhihenbuwa CO. Developing culturally appropriate health programs. In: *Health and culture: beyond the Western paradigm*. London: Sage, 1995, pp. 25–43.

Fadiman A. *The spirit catches you and you fall down: a Hmong child, her American doctors, and the collision of two cultures*. New York: Farrar, Straus and Giroux, 1997.

Greenhalgh T, Helman C, Chowdhury AM. Health beliefs and folk models of diabetes in British Bangladeshis: a qualitative study. *BMJ* 1998;**316**:978–83.

Kelleher D, Hillier S. *Researching cultural differences in health*. London: Routledge, 1996.

Kelleher D, Islam S. The problem of integration: Asian people and diabetes. *J R Soc Med* 1994;**87**: 414–17.

Sheikh A, Gatrad AR. *Caring for Muslim patients*. Oxford: Radcliffe Medical Press, 2000.

Skultans V. Anthropology and narrative. In: Greenhalgh T, Hurwitz B, eds. *Narrative based medicine: dialogue and discourse in clinical practice*. London: BMJ Publications, 1998, pp. 225–32.

The story of Mrs K

Mrs K is 63 years old. Three years ago she was diagnosed with diabetes after she moved to the UK. Her diabetes is tablet controlled. Mrs K was generally accepting of her diabetes but took her tablets irregularly. When the diabetic symptoms returned she would panic and start taking her tablets regularly. Then after a while the "irregularity" returned. Mrs K somehow felt that consistency was not required – perhaps expecting the tablet to "cure" her. Also a strong reason for her attitude was that she felt "old" and it didn't matter any more because life was "practically over". Mrs K's attitude is still the same and she is unshaken in the belief that she is too old.

Why did you choose this story?

It explains some people's attitudes to medication and perhaps the link between age and attitude.

Could anything have been done differently?

Mrs K needed someone to explain that the tablets don't "cure" the diabetes and need to be taken consistently. She needed someone to talk to her about improving her quality of life and that she wasn't too old to care!

What questions or issues does this story raise?

Age plays a part in people's attitude to diabetes.

What are the learning points?

The issue of age needs to be addressed in some way, and that no matter how long you live you can certainly improve your quality of life.

The story of Mr I

A 65-year-old diabetic patient went to Saudi Arabia to do the Haj. Mr I is insulin dependent, and when he went to Mecca he took his insulin and all his medication. But when he got there and after a few days, he thought "I have come to Mecca and I will recover from my problems". He thought he wouldn't need to use insulin any more because he was in a special place. So he stopped taking his insulin. Then after two weeks he had a stroke which left him permanently paralysed. The people who were with Mr I at the time took him to the hospital. But they were friends and not family (and didn't know about his diabetes).

Could anything have been done differently?

It would have been different if there was someone close to him who could have advised Mr I and supported him in taking his insulin and reminded him of his situation.

What questions or issues does this story raise?
Mr I should have understood the diabetes better, and how important insulin is and what it does for your health.

What are the learning points?
- There is a lot to learn about diabetes and how insulin works.
- Mr I should have seen the diabetic nurse before he went to Mecca so he could get a lot of information about being diabetic and travelling.

Tutor's comment
These two stories show how "cultural" beliefs and perceptions can influence compliance with medication. The narrator correctly suggests that a change in expectation of quality of life might be the key to improving the first patient's compliance. Paradoxically, the holy pilgrimage is a common cause of problems in Muslim people with diabetes. A planned pre-travel visit to a diabetes doctor or nurse, with a health advocate or interpreter in attendance, is essential to prevent tragedies like that of Mr I.

The story of Mrs M
Mrs M went to the GP with her father-in-law because her husband was at work. The GP assumed the father-in-law was her husband. Mrs M had to rely on her father-in-law to translate for her. She was too embarrassed to speak about personal matters to her GP in front of her father-in-law and so the GP didn't understand Mrs M's diabetes and the problems she was having with diabetes during her pregnancy. Because the GP did not understand the position Mrs M did not receive appropriate help.

Why did you choose this story?
To highlight how understanding Bengali culture can make a difference.

Could anything have been done differently?
A health advocate would have realised the problems and could have asked the father-in-law to leave the room and translate for Mrs M. The GP should have asked what relationship there was between Mrs M and the man accompanying her. The GP should have had an awareness about Bangladeshi culture and how it could affect Mrs M's communication.

What questions or issues does this story raise?
That culture plays a part and needs to be understood by health professionals.

What are the learning points?
Health advocates are a very important asset.

Tutor's comment
This story is one of many we heard in our group about incorrect assumptions made by doctors about the beliefs, practices or relationships of their Bangladeshi patients. The message seems to be: make fewer assumptions, and enlist the help of a trained advocate.

Unit 9
Educating and supporting other health professionals

Background

Diabetes care is inherently multidisciplinary. The specialist team of nurses, doctors, dieticians, and chiropodists interfaces with the primary health care team, pharmacists, social services, family planning services, advocacy and interpreting services, and lay and voluntary groups. To ensure seamless care, that is, care in which the patient does not suffer from failure of communication across a professional or organisational boundary, we must understand and value one another's roles and responsibilities and provide mutual on-the-job education and support.

Suggested aim for this session

For participants to explore the different roles and responsibilities of different professionals involved in diabetes care, and the implications of these for patient care.

Suggested learning objectives for this session

By the end of this session, participants should be able to:
- give a basic account of the input of key professional and voluntary sector staff to the care of a person with diabetes
- describe a patient whose complex needs require input from several different health and social care staff
- identify potential barriers to seamless care across different professional and organisational interfaces and suggest ways of overcoming these barriers.

Suggestions for group exercises

When you have read the stories in this unit of Mrs Alom and Ms Ali, try one or more of the following:

1. Share further stories of patients whose care was inadequately managed across a professional or organisational boundary. For example, you might have examples in your group of:
   - a patient who was told one thing by the nurse or doctor at the specialist clinic and another by the practice nurse or GP
   - a patient who needed to see a dietician or chiropodist but was not referred or even informed about the service

- a patient who could have benefited from lay or voluntary groups but was not referred to these (see also the example of this on p. 39)
- a patient who was seeing a conventional doctor as well as an alternative practitioner and getting different treatment from each.

2. Consider the issue of "seamless care". The stories on pp. 56 and 57, and perhaps other stories you have shared in your group, are highly emotionally charged because different professionals tend to get frustrated with one another's different world view. Of course, we would all like to see it achieved in practice, but what are the barriers to a truly seamless service? Consider, for example, the following general headings:
   - Professional culture (do some groups have to "know their place"?)
   - Physical proximity (do some teams work in a different building?)
   - Time (is someone always too busy to speak to you?)
   - Personal issues (do some people simply not like each other?)

3. If you have not yet had a go at exercise 2 on p. 42, try it now.

Suggested assignment

Write a short essay with the title "Improving care across boundaries" which is based on one of the stories you have discussed in your group. Suggest three ways in which communication across interprofessional or professional–voluntary sector boundaries could improve. What are the barriers to implementing your suggestions in practice?

Further reading

A guide to roles and responsibilities of health professionals in diabetes

MacKinnon M. *Providing diabetes care in general practice: a practical guide for the primary health care team*, 4th edition. London: Class Publishing, 2002. See ch. 1, "Responsibilities of those involved in the provision of diabetes care", pp. 1–12.

Books about linkworking and multidisciplinary care

Gorman P. *Managing multidisciplinary teams in the NHS*. London: Kogan Page, 1998.

Levinson R, Gillam S. *Linkworkers in primary care*. London: King's Fund, 1998.

Pritchard P, Pritchard J. *Teamwork for primary and shared care: a practical workbook*, 2nd edition. Oxford: Oxford Medical Publications, 1994.

The story of Mrs Alom

Mrs Alom has been suffering from diabetes for five years. She is a 45-year-old housewife. She is on diabetic tablets and on blood pressure tablets. Her asthma has been very bad and she is trying very hard to lose weight. The GP she saw yesterday told her that she needs to lose weight and her diabetes is out of control. He did not explain to her clearly about her sugar level being high. Mrs Alom also forgot to mention that she has not been taking her diabetes tablets for 3 days because they have finished. Mrs Alom was very upset. She did not understand why her sugar level was high, also she kept saying that she is seeing a dietician for her weight and is doing exercise to help her lose weight.

I [health advocate] saw Mrs Alom in the waiting room and asked her what was wrong. After explaining I went and told her GP that she was not taking her tablets because they had run out. The GP was very angry, but I mentioned to him that Mrs Alom had a lot of problems and he should understand and be sympathetic towards her instead of shouting to her.

Why did you choose this story?

Mrs Alom also suffers from asthma, is overweight and has high blood pressure.

Could anything have been done differently?

The GP should have booked Mrs Alom with an advocate and also understood that a patient suffering from so many illnesses would sometimes make mistakes if she doesn't understand clearly. Also Mrs Alom needs to have the repeat prescription system explained so she does not run out of medicine.

What questions or issues does this story raise?

- More explaining of how to take medicines
- What to do if medication finishes, especially if patients suffers from diabetes, blood pressure, asthma, etc.
- GPs should understand that a client may become upset if issues regarding overweight are not talked about sympathetically.

What are the learning points?

- A health advocate should have been present.
- Clients may need more information on the health services system.
- People who have a weight problem should be told about diet more carefully, as explanations may be offensive.

This story really upset me because I saw how upset Mrs Alom was. I made sure all her future appointments were booked when I was present, to avoid any future misunderstandings.

Tutor's comment

See next story

The story of Ms Ali

Ms Ali attended her local health clinic to find out the results of her tests, due to the symptoms she was having, which she thought might be due to diabetes. When she went to hear the results a Bengali health advocate was present to translate and told her that her kidneys had "gone bad", when in fact she just had a kidney infection. Ms Ali interpreted "gone bad" to mean kidney failure and became very upset.

Ms Ali was very distressed thinking her kidneys had failed. She only reacted emotionally after leaving the clinic, as beforehand she was too shocked by the news. She went to the One Stop Health Shop at a local community centre where she burst into tears and told a Bengali nurse what had happened, in Bengali. The nurse contacted the GP straight away who reassured her and told her to tell Ms Ali that it was only a kidney infection. Ms Ali was both angry (with the advocate) and relieved to hear the news.

Why did you choose this story?

To show the lack of communication and training for advocacy workers with regard to medical terminology. Mistakes can make problems seem worse than they really are for the client.

Could anything have been done differently?

The health advocate should have received training in medical terminology based on the relevant health field in which she was working.

What questions or issues does this story raise?

Health advocates act as communicators (a bridge) between health professionals and clients, hence it is vital that they are trained in all aspects of health advocacy beforehand.

What are the learning points?

- Just because a health advocate can speak the same language as the client does not mean he/she is communicating and passing on messages from the professionals to the client accurately.
- In a real life situation the health professional relies solely on the health advocate to pass on information correctly, therefore the role of the health advocate is very important.

Tutor's comment

This story, and the previous one, highlight the contrasting problems when doctors try to do without advocates and when advocates assume too much medical knowledge. The real mistake of both of these health professionals was to assume they were capable of doing a job they were not trained to do. In both cases the person who suffered was the patient.

Unit 10
Diabetes and women's health

Background
Some of the complications of diabetes (such as recurrent thrush or urinary infections) are of an intimate nature and women may not volunteer their symptoms. Many will prefer (and some require) a female doctor or nurse for these aspects of their care.

Diabetes affects contraceptive choices, fertility, and the outcome of pregnancy. One common form of diabetes, gestational diabetes, only occurs during pregnancy. Some ethnic groups (especially south Asians) have a very high incidence of gestational diabetes. Women who have had gestational diabetes are at high risk of developing type 2 diabetes later in life.

If a woman with diabetes does not have very good control in the three months before conception and during pregnancy, the risk of miscarriage and fetal malformation is greatly increased. A poorly controlled diabetic mother may produce an overweight baby who has trouble passing through the birth canal and requires special care in the days following birth. For these reasons, a crucial goal in the young woman with diabetes is to ensure that all pregnancies are optimally planned and that close liaison occurs between all teams and organisations involved in care (including primary health care, family planning clinics, obstetric services, specialist diabetes services, and voluntary groups).

Suggested aim for this session
For participants to explore the experiences, values, and choices of diabetic women around contraception, pregnancy, and other aspects of women's health.

Suggested learning objectives for this session
By the end of this session, participants should be able to:
- give a basic account of how diabetes affects women's health and life choices
- empathise with a patient whose contraceptive choices, fertility, or the outcome of pregnancy were compromised because of diabetes
- identify potential barriers to optimum pregnancy outcome in women with particular needs (for example, those who speak little English) and suggest ways of overcoming these barriers.

Suggestions for group exercises

Read the stories on pp. 61–63, and see also the story of Mrs Iqbal on p. 9, Mrs S on p. 14, and Mrs M on p. 52. When you have done this, try one or more of the following:

1. Share some additional stories of your own about women's health and pregnancy outcome. Find out in particular if anyone in your group has experience of caring for a woman who had any of the following:
   - Problems she was too embarrassed to discuss with the doctor or nurse
   - a sexually transmitted disease
   - difficulty finding a suitable form of contraception
   - difficulty achieving good control before or during pregnancy
   - difficulty getting pregnant
   - serious complications in pregnancy, such as stillbirth or malformation
   - traumatic labour
   - postnatal depression.

2. Role-play a situation in which a woman with diabetes has recently married and wishes to start a family. She has been told by her doctors not to get pregnant until she has lost weight and controlled her diabetes better. But she is desperate for a baby and her in-laws are keen to see a grandchild. When you have done the role-play, ask those who played the different people to say how they felt. What measures do you think health professionals should adopt to support women to plan their pregnancies optimally?

3. Consider the needs of a particular group of patients (for example, from a particular ethnic minority or a hard-to-reach group such as adolescents who have defaulted from routine diabetes follow-up). Discuss what their overall needs are as a group, and make some specific suggestions for adapting the service in your area to meet those needs. Pay particular attention to communication across professional and organisational boundaries and about how your suggestions would be made to work in practice.

Suggested assignment

Write up any of the stories discussed above, listing five main learning points. Imagine your essay will be used as part of a training pack about women's health for a predominantly male group of doctors with little understanding of this particular culture. You will therefore need to emphasise both the needs and perspective of women in general, and also the particular cultural and religious needs of your chosen patient.

Further reading

Books on women's health issues for health professionals

Schott J, Henley A. *Culture, religion and childbearing in a multi-racial society – a handbook for health professionals.* Oxford: Butterworth–Heinemann, 1996.

Sheikh A, Gatrad AR. *Caring for Muslim patients.* Oxford: Radcliffe Medical Press, 2000.

Health guides for women with diabetes

Various leaflets on women's health available free from Diabetes UK (see p. 8 for details).

Szarewski A, Guillebaud J. *Contraception – a users' handbook.* Oxford: Oxford University Press, 2001.

Diabetes UK website – for professionals and the public

http://www.diabetes.org.uk/

The story of Mrs Nessa

Mrs Nessa is a 32-year-old housewife who has three children. She started to suffer from diabetes after her second child and was diet controlled. During her fourth pregnancy she was referred again to the diabetic clinic for assessment. Her diet was not helping her so she was told about insulin injections. The baby was getting big, her sugar levels were high and she was feeling unwell. She wasn't keeping good records either and when she came for her appointment her blood test showed higher than normal.

Mrs Nessa should have been monitoring her blood sugar properly and needed to see someone. She didn't know much about diabetes, what it could do to her baby or how it could affect her. Finally, Mrs Nessa was admitted to hospital. She was shown how to give the insulin to get her sugar levels controlled but she was still confused and not drawing up the insulin.

Why did you choose this story?

Although Mrs Nessa knew about diabetes she was still confused about insulin injections and was frightened.

Could anything have been done differently?

Mrs Nessa should have stayed in hospital until she knew how to give her insulin and she should have been shown by an advocate who spoke her language. When discharged from hospital one of the nurses should have done a home visit and checked to see Mrs Nessa was giving herself the right amount of insulin and recording her blood sugars.

What questions or issues does this story raise?

Mrs Nessa was frightened of the injection because she knew she had to give it to herself and she also thought she would be on insulin for the rest of her life.

What are the learning points?

People like Mrs Nessa need to go to sessions where they can talk to other people with diabetes. She could also be told that she may not need insulin after she has had the baby.

Tutor's comment

This story shows that even women who have had diabetes for some time can become confused and anxious when efforts to control the diabetes are stepped up during pregnancy. Women who are tablet controlled are routinely changed to insulin during pregnancy because of a theoretical risk that diabetic tablets may damage the fetus. Even diet controlled diabetic women may need to start insulin temporarily in pregnancy. Like Mrs Nessa, they may find this change difficult and may wrongly think that the insulin will have to be continued after the baby is born.

The story of Mrs Begum

Mrs Begum is now 48 years old. She lives with her four children and developed diabetes after having her first child. Mrs Begum has a family history of diabetes. Her father, grandfather, and uncles all suffer with this problem. Mrs Begum developed diabetes during her first pregnancy. Her diet was not very well controlled and slowly her diabetes was getting higher. She ended up having insulin and was admitted to hospital because her sugars were not well controlled even though she was on insulin.

Mrs Begum was getting worried that she might have a too-big baby. She could not have a "normal" delivery and this was a major worry for her. The doctor told her that if the baby is getting too big it is best for her to have a caesarean and it is safe for the baby.

Could anything have been done differently?

While Mrs Begum was in hospital she was told how to give herself insulin. She was still confused, however, and the midwife used to give her the injections. Mrs Begum needed support and needed time to get used to insulin injections.

What questions or issues does this story raise?

While Mrs Begum was given insulin her sugars came slowly under control. Afterwards she learnt how to give herself injections. She knew how important it was to give insulin and that if her sugars were well controlled the baby might be the right size and she might not need a caesarean.

Tutor's comment

The desire to give birth "naturally" may stem from a simple wish to avoid "medicalising" the birth, but there may be additional religious or cultural beliefs about treatment of the child's soul or the need to clear body fluids adequately through the proper channels. But obstetric management should not be compromised by misplaced respect for religious and cultural traditions. As this narrator suggests, Mrs Begum is ill-informed and frightened, and her chief need is for sensitive explanation of the various medical risks and options. A non-judgemental counselling and education programme before the onset of pregnancy should have enabled her to link her desire (for a normal baby born by the normal route) with the means to that end (intensive management of her diabetes with insulin therapy), and to gain the skills and confidence to achieve this with the help of the diabetes specialist nurse.

The story of Mrs Q

Mrs Q, a 34-year-old housewife, is 4 months pregnant and a diabetic. When she was 2 months pregnant she was bleeding so she thought she was having a miscarriage. She came for a check-up two weeks ago and the doctor wanted to confirm that she was still pregnant and sent her for a scan. The scan result showed that she is 16+ weeks pregnant. Mrs Q did not want to keep the baby as she is diabetic and when she was previously pregnant she was in and out of hospital and had to go on insulin. At the moment she has also stopped taking her diabetic medication.

Mrs Q was very upset. She had thought she had lost the baby and was relieved, as she had decided to have a termination if she was pregnant again. Now she is worried sick as she is over 4 months pregnant and over the normal 12 weeks to have a termination. Her doctor realised she was very upset and read from her notes about her previous pregnancy and saw that she did suffer a lot and was very unwell. Her doctor decided to refer her for counselling and a termination.

Why did you choose this story?
I felt very sad about Mrs Q's situation and decided to help her overcome some of her problems.

Could anything have been done differently?
Mrs Q should have seen her doctor when she started bleeding at 2 months so she could have been referred there and then.

What questions or issues does this story raise?
Many clients are not aware of the facilities provided by the NHS or health centres.

What are the learning points?
More health promotion work should be done and information given out to patients so that they know what services are available to them.

Tutor's comment
It is often assumed that Muslim patients never wish to have a termination of pregnancy. But whilst beliefs and attitudes towards termination are influenced to a large extent by religious and cultural norms, they are also modified by individual preference – which, as in this case, is often profoundly influenced by past experience. Mrs Q found her previous pregnancy on insulin frightening and traumatic, and had already decided not to go through it again. But she did not know that bleeding in early pregnancy does not always mean a miscarriage. Her doctor managed to determine, and support, her personal choice even at the late stage of presentation. As this narrator correctly concludes, women from minority ethnic groups would benefit from sensitive health promotion before, during, and after their pregnancies.

Appendix
Template for writing up a story

We were initially reluctant to offer any form of template lest this be seen as the "correct" structure for telling a story or for drawing learning points from it. However, we found that some group members valued a loose structure to help them formulate their stories, and the group discussions that were held around those stories, into meaningful elements of learning. The template overleaf is intended to be adapted (or abandoned!) as needed.

There are five key features to the template, which we feel are important to gaining the maximum educational value from each story. Compare this list of features with the defining characteristics of a story as described on p. ix and with the educational value of small group work on p. xvi (and in particular the Figure on p. xix).

- The story focuses on an **individual patient or client** and not on a disease, a part of the body, a drug, or some other "biomedical" perspective. It is told from the viewpoint of that person and includes what is relevant to him or her.
- There is a **plot**, that is, the story begins; things happen; we see what emerges. The narrative form suggests both meaning and causality to the unfolding of events (for example, "The doctor told him he had diabetes and he became depressed" suggests that he became depressed *as a result of* the news).
- The story explicitly includes a description of the **feelings and emotions** of key characters. A patient given the news that they need insulin might be angry, confused, or frightened; each of these different emotions would influence the behaviour of the other characters and the best strategy for a positive outcome. A deliberate focus on the patient's (and the health professional's) emotions often highlights differences in perspective and particular failures in understanding and communication.
- The narrator is invited to **reflect on** the story and construct an alternative ending ("Should anything have been done differently?").
- The narrator is invited to **draw out learning points** for their own learning and professional practice.

This template is designed primarily for the health professional who, like the people in our own learning group, tells a story about a patient or client. There are some similarities with Kleinman's focus on the patient's own story, which he suggests can be prompted via eight questions:[1]

- What do you call the problem?
- What do you think has caused it?
- Why do you think it started when it did?
- What do you think the sickness does – and how?
- How severe do you think it is?
- What problems has it caused?
- What kind of treatment do you think you should get, and what are the most important results it will produce?
- What do you fear most about the condition?

In our more recent research with interorganisational groups addressing service level issues, we have modified the last question in our template ("What are the learning points for you or other people?") to a more service-oriented question ("What are the points for the design and development of services in this area?"). We plan to test our "service development" template further and to publish a separate study on this dimension of storytelling.

Reference

1 Kleinman A. *The illness narratives: suffering, healing and the human condition.* New York: Basic Books, 1988.

Name

Storytelling template

Who is the story about? *(e.g. Mrs J.P. – a 53-year-old housewife)*

....

Why have you chosen this story?

....
....

What happened in the story? *(continue on the back of this page if necessary)*

....
....
....
....
....
....
....
....
....
....

How did the people in the story feel or react?

....
....
....
....
....
....

What was the outcome?

....
....
....
....
....

Should anything have been done differently, and if so, what and how?

....

....

....

....

....

....

What questions or issues does this story raise?

....

....

....

....

....

What are the learning points for you and for other people?

....

....

....

....

....

....

Any other comments?

....

....

....

....

Signed:	Date:

For course organiser
What would help the learner(s) meet the learning needs identified here?

....

....

....

....

....

Index

Page numbers in **bold** refer to figures: those in *italics* refer to tables or boxed materials.